THE COMPLETE PROSTATE BOOK

Prostate problems are no longer thought of as an 'old man's disease'. A recent study of Mathews Foundation for Prostate Cancer Research, USA, reports that in reality 20 per cent of the victims are under the age of sixty five and a startling number are only in their forties ...

Prostate problems are treatable. Early detection is crucial in providing proper treatment for controlling the problem. No one enjoys pain, but in the case of prostate, pain is often a blessing in disguise: it provides an early warning to see a physician and to resolve the problem quickly.

Prostate problems are preventable. Often people and their families suffer for not knowing this important truth. Developing a balanced lifestyle is vital. A lifestyle of adequate exercise, low-fat diet, minimal consumption of alcohol, cutting out cigarettes, and learning to manage stress — all controllable factors — can substantially improve chances of a full and healthy life.

This comprehensive, authoritative, and friendly book discusses prevention and up to date treatment options, both non-surgical and surgical, including emerging therapies, for prostate problems. It answers directly the concern all men have for prostate health and other related issues.

AF647392

Health Care in
Orient Paperbacks

The Asthma Self-Help Book
The Walking Diet
Conquering Backpain
Overcoming Migraines and Other Headaches
Preventing Heart Disease: Exercising for a Healthy Heart
Homoeopathic Remedies for Middle and Old Age
The Complete Book of Family Homoeopathic Medicine
Home Guide to Medical Emergencies

To Joan Ellen Belshin, who has tolerated my type A behavior for forty-five years and who, with my sons Joseph, Matthew, and daughter Maryann Spiegelman, have given me the love and inspiration to complete this project.

To my grandchildren, Sarah and Daniel, my future grandchildren, and all children throughout the world. I'm hopeful that the medical researchers who work diligently to uncover the unknowns of chronic diseases will make major breakthroughs for future generations.

Acknowledgments

This book has been made possible by the support and encouragement of many individuals in the medical profession and related fields.

Special thanks to Ralph de Vere White, M.D., chairman of the department of urology at the University of California at Davis, who took a great deal of time from his research and educational activities to provide valued counsel and guidance.

Mary Lou Wright, executive director of the Mathews Foundation for Prostate Cancer Research, and KD Proffit, M.I.S., at the Sutter Health Resource Center, and the staff librarians at the University of California at Davis were most helpful in providing me with a variety of publications and research pertaining to benign prostatic hyperplasia and prostate cancer.

THE COMPLETE PROSTATE BOOK

Lee Belshin, M.S.

Foreword by Ralph deVere White, M.D.,
Chairman, Department of Urology
University of California

Written in Cooperation
with the Mathews Foundation for
Prostate Cancer Research

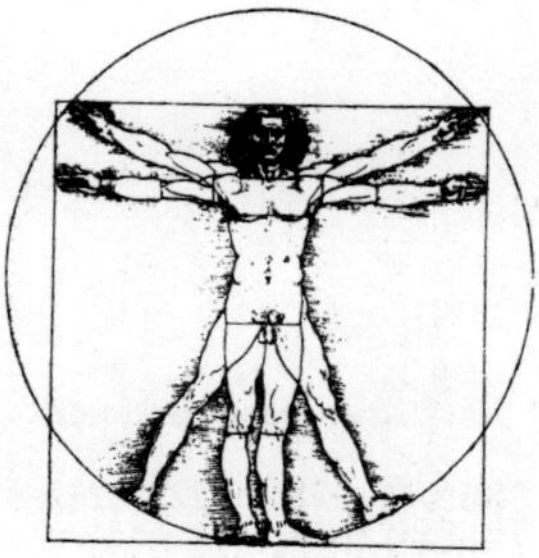

Orient Paperbacks
DELHI | MUMBAI | HYDERABAD

Disclaimer

This book is not intended to replace medical guidance. Persons under doctor's care for prostate-related health problems should consult with their physicians. Responsibility for any adverse effects resulting from the use of information in this book rests solely with the reader.

All rights reserved. No part of this publication may be reproduced or transmitted in any form or by any means, electronic or mechanical, including photocopying and recording, or introduced into any information storage and retrieval system without the written permission of the copyright owner and the publisher of this book. Brief quotations may be used in reviews prepared for inclusion in a magazine, newspaper, or broadcast.

www.orientpaperbacks.com

ISBN 13: 978-81-222-0252-6
ISBN 10: 81-222-0252-7

1st Published in Orient Paperbacks 1999

The Complete Prostate Book: Every Man's Guide

© 1997, Lee Belshin

Cover design by Vision Studio

Published in arrangement with
Prima Communications, Inc.

Published by
Orient Paperbacks
(A division of Vision Books Pvt. Ltd.)
5A/8 Ansari Road, New Delhi-110 002

Printed in India at
Ravindra Printing Press, Delhi-110 006

Contents

III

What to Do If You Have Prostate Cancer

IV

Surgery

V

A Lifestyle for a Healthy Prostate

VI

On the Horizon

Foreword

How time has changed! A few years ago, you could search in the best bookstores in the country and rarely find anything written on the subject of the prostate. Today, many bookstores carry a wide variety of books written about various prostate problems.

Regrettably, the subject's popularity indicates that people's interest in this gland goes beyond just another fashionable topic in the book circle. You may ask, *why should I choose this book over others?* Speaking from my twenty-five years of experience as a urologist, I think Mr. Belshin brings about a most unique perspective on the subject to his readers.

Mr. Belshin has previously published an extremely well-read and popular book dealing with cardiovascular problems. He now brings the same insight to the prostate, reviewing many of the problems that the prostate can inflict on the unsuspecting male population. After reading this book, you can learn to take some of the proper steps to preventing prostate disease. Unlike many others who have written on the subject, Mr. Belshin has a first-hand knowledge of prostate problems since he had personally dealt with benign enlargement of the gland.

This book discusses the slow growth and diagnosis of prostate cancer and views the disease as an overall health problem rather than solely a prostate problem. In this regard, the book will offer much information regarding diet, exercise, and stress management, and is an overall reference guide on male health issues.

Finally, Mr. Belshin has unique abilities to entertain and inform at the same time. In many ways, this book can be seen as the first novel in which the prostate plays a starring role!

Read, enjoy, and be informed!

Ralph W. deVere White, M.D.
Professor and chairman, Department of Urology
University of California at Davis, School of Medicine

Introduction

The first authentic written description of the prostate gland was given by Niccolo Massa, a Venetian physician who died in 1563. It was a century later, in 1649, before another Italian physician, Biolanus, suggested that the prostate could obstruct the passage of urine.

The word "prostate" is derived from both Greek and Latin words meaning "standing before." Those of you who, like me, have suffered from benign prostatic hyperplasia (BPH) may feel that it aptly describes the time we spend standing before the urinal. In fact, I was tempted to title this book *To Pee or Not To Pee.*

Today, disorders of the prostate gland are fast becoming the most disturbing, costly, and bewildering health problem of the nineties. By the age of sixty, over 50 percent of men will suffer from BPH, an enlargement of the prostate gland; by the age of eighty-five, that number rises to 85 percent. In addition, it is predicted that in 1996 over 244,000 American men will be diagnosed with prostate cancer, and more than forty thousand will die from it—a more than 110 percent increase over the last ten years.

Yet until recently, most men have known little about their prostate glands. Bob Dole expressed his astonishment and dismay when he was diagnosed in 1991 as having cancer of the prostate: "I was, like most men, barely aware that it could develop into a life-threatening problem."

The purpose of this book is to help the more than 50 percent of American men who will develop problems of the prostate, whether it be prostatitis, benign prostatic hyperplasia, or prostate cancer. I will introduce you to information that may help you to prevent prostate problems, and I will discuss how to treat and defeat any problems that may arise so that you can lead a healthier, happier life.

Interestingly, according to a recent study, some segments of our population are more at risk than others. For example, the danger of prostate hypertrophy is higher in Jewish men than among Protestants and Catholics, and higher in African-Americans than in Caucasians. African-Americans have, by far, the highest prostate cancer rate in the world; their risk is 40 percent higher than that of Caucasians. The incidence of prostate cancer is relatively low in the South America, China, Japan, the Philippines, and parts of Africa; incidence is relatively high in North America and Europe. Hispanic men appear to blessed with a high degree of protection against prostate cancer. The only other mammalian species that suffers from benign enlargement of the prostate is man's best friend, his dog.

I felt moved to write this book because, as a public health educator, a teacher of gerontology, and an insurance executive, I have observed too many needless deaths. Often people die because their lifestyle involves insufficient exercise, a high-fat diet, too many cigarettes, and an inability to manage stress—all controllable factors.

Seeing so much preventable loss of life first motivated me to write two books on preventing coronary artery disease: *Love Your Heart* and *Love Your Heart Guide for the 1990's*. While doing research for these books, I was amazed at the similarity of causes that contribute to a fatal heart attack and to prostate cancer.

GROWING AWARENESS OF PROSTATE PROBLEMS

Not long ago, men rarely talked about prostate problems, but with the graying of America, the prostate is becoming impossible to ignore. I have yet to play in a golf foursome without seeing at least one player excuse himself several times to visit the men's room.

Interruptions during a tennis foursome are usually not only to resolve a close line call, but for a male player to rush to the lavatory.

Fortunately, prostate problems are now being discussed openly. Famous Americans from Bob Dole to retired general Norman Schwartzkopf, Buffalo Bills football coach Marv Levy, and junk bond king Michael Milken have openly discussed their bouts with prostate cancer. Milken and others are encouraging men to get tested and to discover the disease early, when it is most treatable. Recently on CNN, Larry King and a panel of prominent urologists and celebrities had a heart-to-heart chat about the impact that prostate disorders had on their lives, giving the issue much-needed publicity.

At one time, admitting to having prostate cancer would have meant the end of one's career, especially for a politician seeking higher office. But there is nothing shameful about the disease except the neglect of so many males who do not get tested for it. The more you understand about prostate cancer, the better your odds are of overcoming it.

It is also important to remember that prostate problems are treatable. Death is not inevitable, as the majority of males fear. In fact, many doctors will tell you that if you have to be afflicted by a form of cancer, prostate cancer is the one to choose; it is slow-growing, and many males live out their lives without even knowing that they have it. More men will die with the disease than of the disease.

PART I

The Basics

CHAPTER ONE

The Prostate Gland

The prostate gland is situated just below the bladder and surrounding the urethra in the male reproductive system. It is firm and is often likened in shape to an apple with its core removed.

Medical scientists are not fully aware of the prostate's function, but we do know that it adds vital nutrients and fluid to assist in sex and reproduction. The prostate is referred to as an accessory sex gland: its function is sexual, but it is only indirectly involved in procreation. The prostate gland produces a lubricant that helps move sperm through the body and onward in its mission to fertilize an egg. The fluid serves as a vehicle in which the spermatozoa can travel at the time of ejaculation. Prostatic fluid also provides nourishment to the spermatozoa so that they can live after ejaculation and continue on their journey.

The prostate gland manufactures fluid continuously and stores it, so the fluid will be ready to perform its role again and again. Another vital function of this gland is to act as a valve that allows sperm and urine to flow in the right direction.

LIVING WITH THE PROSTATE

When a male baby is born, his prostate gland is about the size of the tip of an adult's little finger. The gland grows slowly during the first thirty years of life to reach its full size, which is about the

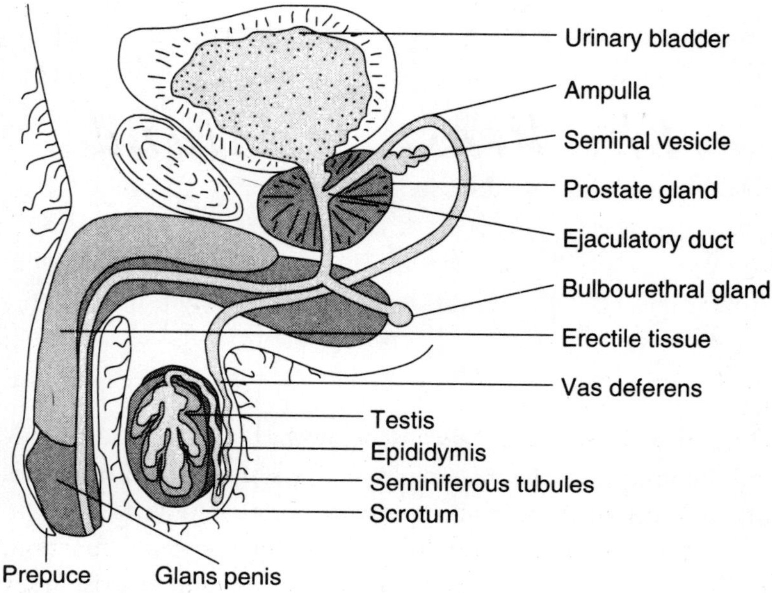

THE MALE REPRODUCTIVE SYSTEM

size and shape of a large chestnut or occasionally even that of a grapefruit. (In this area, bigger is not better.)

Although physicians are not fully aware of the prostate's function, they do know that it adds vital nutrients and fluid to the sperm. The gland produces a lubricant which helps move sperm through the body, and onward in its mission to fertilize an egg. Prostatic fluid also provides nourishment to the spermatozoa so that they can live after ejaculation and continue on their vital journey.

The size of the prostate gland alone does not determine the amount of grief it will cause. If the capsule (the fibrous outlining of the prostate) is firm and exerts compression on the urethral tube (the tube that carries urine or semen out of the body), it will cause symptoms even if the prostate not very large.

The early growth of a young man's prostate gland may unexpectedly give an abrupt wake-up call—literally. It causes him to awaken often during the night with a sudden urge to urinate (a condition called nocturia). Then, if getting up from a warm, cozy bed isn't bad enough, when he gets to the bathroom, very little happens. And when the hesitant stream finally moves, it comes out as a dribble—a definite sign that an enlarged prostate is putting a stranglehold on his urethra.

Picture the urethra as a garden hose that you hold in your hand. If you squeeze the hose, the water will dribble out; if you apply more pressure, no water will flow. A similar effect is caused by the prostate gland. As it enlarges, both inward and upward, it compresses the urethra and prevents a smooth flow of urine.

An enlarged prostate not only can keep a man from getting a decent night's sleep, but also can irritate him in the workplace. He may continuously feel that he has to empty his bladder (the organ where urine is stored), and as soon as he returns from an unsuccessful attempt to do so, he may feel an immediate need to go right back and try again—not a very pleasant way to spend the day (his associates may even start to speculate as to why he is constantly rushing off to the lavatory).

Men who have to travel for business may find prostate enlargement even more disrupting. I developed benign prostatic hyperplasia (BPH) just as I was hired by a national investment firm to present a series of training sessions in twenty-six states. During the tour, I constantly feared that I would have to excuse myself from the lectern in the middle of a speech. Fortunately, this did not happen, but it created additional pressure for me, not only while talking but also while traveling. I actually carried an empty bottle just in case.

THE ONSET OF PROSTATE PROBLEMS

Prostate problems are thought of as an "old man's disease," but this is not the case. Mary Lou Wright, Executive Director of the

Mathews Foundation for Prostate Cancer Research, states, "In reality, at least 20 percent of its victims are under the age of sixty-five. A startling number are only in their forties. For reasons that remain unknown, when this disease strikes younger victims, it seems to occur in a more virulent form. Prostate cancers in older men may grow slowly and produce no symptoms for many years. In younger men, the cancers metastasize (spread from one organ structure to another) more quickly, often spreading to surrounding bone. When that happens, death is often the only prognosis."

Many men in their forties notice a change in their urination, but it is not usually radical enough to alarm them. Later, however, if the urine has an increasingly difficult time traveling through the narrowed passageway, the bladder will have to work harder to push the urine out. This added effort causes the bladder walls to thicken and stretch out of shape. As time passes, the overworked bladder loses its efficiency and some urine may be retained; if untreated, a bladder infection or, in extreme cases, kidney failure may develop.

No one enjoys pain, but in the case of the prostate, pain can be a blessing in disguise: it provides an early warning to see a physician and hopefully resolve the problem at an early stage.

Early detection is crucial in providing proper treatment for cancer of the prostate. Perhaps less than a third of prostate cancers are found early enough to respond to treatment. Since approximately one out of every ten American men develop prostate cancer and more than 41,000 die annually from this disease, it is not something to ignore.

MYTHS ABOUT THE PROSTATE GLAND

As with most medical problems, there are many myths and unjustified fears to dispel. Let us look at the facts regarding some of the false notions about the prostate gland.

Myth #1: Too much or too little sexual activity is the main cause of prostate disorders

I can see a lot of men rushing to share this myth with their sexual partners. The notion does have a bit of merit. Prostate congestion (or prostatostasis)—an enlargement of the prostate gland with prostate secretions, which urologists attribute to irregular or infrequent orgasms and ejaculation—was at one time labeled "priest's disease," as it was common among men who did not masturbate or have sexual intercourse. Similar problems occur with many teenagers who delay ejaculation during intercourse or masturbation; this practice disrupts the natural bodily rhythms and irritates the prostate. Most physicians agree that it is better to complete the sexual act to prevent congestion. The most common way to bring on prostate congestion is to engage in extended sexual stimulation and then stop without ejaculating.

Prostate congestion is not a typical problem among younger men. Nocturnal emissions (wet dreams), masturbation, and the availability of willing partners usually help them to avoid prostate congestion. But among the older population, this is a more common problem. As the tendency for sexual activity diminishes, the incidence of prostate cancer increases.

On the other hand, a high level of sexual activity in a short period of time can also aggravate the prostate gland. Men who try to be sexual giants and to set records in this category are putting themselves at risk.

Having a normal, healthy sex life is the best way to prevent many problems, including prostate disorders; as in so many other fields, moderation is the healthiest choice.

Myth #2: Prostate surgery will make a man impotent, incontinent, or both

You will surely hear a story sooner or later about a poor soul who went into the hospital to relieve the symptoms of BPH or to stop the growth of prostate cancer and came out less of a man; the cure was worse than the problem. There is some risk that problems will occur following surgery or treatment for these diseases. However, the danger is often exaggerated.

There are new and promising treatments for both BPH and prostate cancer that will not put an end to your sex life. In fact, in many cases it will improve. Surgical techniques have evolved that enable a doctor to remove malignant cells without damaging the nerves that are necessary for an erection. If complications do develop, there are many reconstructive devices and other techniques that will enable a man to be sexually active (see Chapter 12).

It is understandable for a man to fear loss of sexual potency, but the fear itself could actually affect his rehabilitation. Any such fears should be openly discussed with a doctor.

Myth #3: A man with BPH will probably develop prostate cancer

Although many patients with BPH do develop prostate cancer, it is not inevitable. Since the symptoms of both conditions are similar, it is important to see a physician when they appear. The symptoms of an enlarged prostate may disguise a growing cancer of the prostate, so if you experience difficult, painful, or burning urination, if you feel the need to urinate frequently, and if you have difficulty in stopping and starting, report these symptoms immediately to your doctor. If it is cancer, the earlier it is detected the better the chance for a cure. If it is BPH, the peace of mind it will give you is well worth the cost of the appointment.

More help may be on the way to address the problems associated with an enlarged prostate. According to George Margolis, a retired medical school professor, "The overall news for treating enlarged prostates is definitely good. We're looking at some of the most rapid changes we've ever seen." New drugs and methods of treatment are now available where not too long ago surgery was the only option.

CHAPTER TWO

Benign Prostatic Hyperplasia and Prostatitis

Symptoms of benign prostatic hyperplasia and prostatitis are the most common reasons for a man to visit his primary-care physician or urologist. It is probably also safe to say that there are no other annoyances that cause more fear or anxiety in a man.

BENIGN PROSTATIC HYPERPLASIA (BPH)

The prostate gland is a perfectly functioning system unless a new kind of tissue, known as adenoma (benign tumor), arises from the normal prostate tissue, signaling the onset of benign prostatic hyperplasia (BPH). This nonmalignant but abnormal cell growth spreads inward as well as outward and enlarges the prostate gland, tightening around the urethra much like a clamp around a hose and thereby reducing the force and size of the urine stream. This problem may begin ten to twenty years before symptoms become apparent.

You may have BPH if you experience increased frequency of urination, a delay in being able to start the stream or stop, and a continuing dribble (or incomplete emptying) of the bladder. Benign prostatic hyperplasia is often referred to as "the curse of aging men." For those who have BPH, gone are the days of more youthful years, when boys participated in contests to demonstrate who had the most powerful flow. As we age, BPH can disrupt the harmony of our life with the constant pit stops required throughout the day and evening.

In addition to the common symptoms of BPH, there are other warning signs: blood or pus in the urine, painful ejaculation, and continuing pain in the lower back, hips, or thighs. It is important to realize that these symptoms may also signify a more serious condition than BPH. Sometimes an enlarged prostate indicates malignant tissue that can spread to other parts of the body (see Chapter 3).

Although BPH is not malignant and does not always develop into a cancerous condition, a man can have both BPH and prostate cancer. Much is still not known about BPH. But one thing is certain: it is related to the presence of the male hormones that are responsible for secondary sex characteristics. That is why male eunuchs, who have had their testicles removed or whose testicles become unusable, do not develop BPH. Jewish men have a higher incidence of BPH than do Protestant or Catholic men. Man's best friend, the dog, is also troubled by BPH.

The good news is that you do not have to suffer from the symptoms of BPH, which have an obvious impact on the quality of your life. It is treatable.

BPH treatment depends on whether the symptoms are unbearable or the urinary function is severely affected. If you have BPH but can adjust to the symptoms, your doctor may very well choose a program referred to as "watchful waiting." This program involves annual (or more frequent) checkups, depending on the individual problem of the patient.

When the problem becomes intolerable, surgery is the preferred choice of physicians at the present time. We will discuss both the nonsurgical and surgical treatments of BPH later in this book.

PROSTATITIS

An enlarged prostate gland might also indicate the presence of prostatitis. Prostatitis is often referred to as Everyman's prostate problem, since it affects thousands of men each year. This infection can be caused by the presence of bacteria. It makes the prostate tissue swell, causing obstruction.

Among male patients, prostatitis accounts for about 25 percent of the visits to a doctor for genitourinary tract complaints. Frequent and painful urination is a common symptom, accompanied by a feeling that the bladder cannot be completely emptied. Pain or aching may be felt in the rectum, the groin, the end of the penis, or the lower back. The infection may cause painful, bloody, or premature ejaculation. Even if pain is not present, in the mornings a small, watery discharge may appear at the tip of the penis; this discharge sometimes causes the opening of the urethra to stick together, or it may stain the inside of a man's shorts. An itching feeling in the penis, pain while defecating, or cloudy urine might also occur—all are good reasons to see a doctor as soon as possible.

There are various types of prostatitis. If you see a doctor for the symptoms described above, the doctor will most likely take a culture of your semen or prostatic secretions to see which of the varieties of prostatitis you have. Obtaining this sample takes only a few seconds. The doctor will bear down on the back wall with his finger and stroke the gland. The pressure will cause a small quantity of fluid to flow out of the gland and into the urethra. The fluid emerges at the tip of the penis and will be collected on a microscope slide to be examined. The laboratory report may indicate that you have one of the following types of prostatitis.

Bacterial Prostatitis

A sudden infusion of bacteria into the gland causes swelling. Symptoms are chills, fever, and a painful and frequent need to urinate. As threatening as it may sound, it can be treated successfully with antibiotics and bed rest. A follow-up visit to the doctor is important to make sure the condition doesn't become chronic.

Chronic Bacterial Prostatitis

This variant can be caused by bacteria that reach the prostate via the rectum or through the bloodstream. Gonorrhea can also cause this problem. Sexual partners are putting themselves at risk of being infected. Often the only symptom is a bladder infection. This condition is treatable with a combination of drugs.

Prostatodynia

Swelling of the prostate without an infection indicates the presence of this annoyance. Many men go to their urologist with this condition, which is about eight times more common than bacterial prostatitis. Doctors are not sure what causes it; despite the presence of inflamed cells, no infectious agent can be found. The condition may result from destruction of the fluid-producing glands within the prostate. This typically happens to a man who, accustomed to ejaculating several times a week, finds that routine suddenly curtailed. The gland fills with fluid, causing inflammation (prostatosis). Prostatodynia is usually relieved by use of hot sitz baths, muscle relaxants, or other drugs.

Prostatostasis

Prostatostasis is a condition in which the prostate becomes congested. Bacteria are not the cause of this problem. In prostatostasis, the prostate produces more fluid than is released by ejaculation. This can result in the enlarged prostate pressing on the urethra and not allowing the bladder to empty. As discussed earlier, if a man does not ejaculate, prostate fluid will build up. The frequency of ejaculation needed to empty the prostate gland is different for each male. Many doctors use prostatic massage to relieve this condition. The doctor inserts his finger as during a digital rectal exam and then forcefully massages each of the two lateral lobes that often grow into the prostatic urethra and cause the symptoms of BPH; secretions come out through the urethra, relieving the pressure.

This sounds like a simple enough therapy, but Dr. Stephen N. Rous, a prominent urologist and author of books on the prostate, refers to the practice as "chronic remunerative prostatitis," because he feels that the massage serves no purpose other than to separate a patient from his money.

A REGIMEN FOR PROSTATITIS SUFFERERS

If you have any form of prostatitis, your physician will probably suggest that you follow a regimen as described below:

1. Avoid caffeine, chocolate, alcohol, pepper, decongestants, APC (Tylenol with coedingeneris), Anacin, and Excedrin. These substances can cause further irritation. Aspirin, Bufferin, and Tylenol are okay.
2. Relieve prostate congestion by ejaculation.
3. Take a hot sitz bath for an hour.
4. Void the bladder at regular intervals; do not over-hold urine.
5. Take zinc in low doses (50 milligrams may be helpful).
6. Drink plenty of fluids.
7. Take stool softeners, if desired, to make bowel movements less painful.

CHAPTER THREE

Prostate Cancer

Prostate cancer strikes 20 percent more men than does lung cancer. It strikes more men than do cancers of the larynx, pancreas, stomach, kidney, mouth, or throat. For a long time, it was the cancer that men did not talk about. To have prostate cancer was considered the ultimate weakness and loss of "machismo."

Fortunately, it is no longer considered shameful to have prostate cancer. Well-known personalities such as former senator Alan Cranston, Supreme Court justices Harry A. Blackman and John Paul Stevens, rock star Frank Zappa, and two-time Nobel Prize winner Linus Pauling have gone public with their prostate cancer stories. In their deaths from prostate cancer, France's Prime Minister François Mitterrand and controversial pop-culture icon Timothy Leary have contributed to public awareness of the condition.

Thanks to publicity and the advent of more effective means of diagnosis and treatment, men are finally talking about prostate cancer. Just as men compare their cholesterol levels over lunch, they are now openly discussing their Prostate-Specific Antigen levels. According to *Cancer Practice* magazine, primary prevention includes risk assessment and health education to facilitate making choices for a healthy lifestyle. Part V of this book will provide you with vital information about preventive lifestyle choices, such as exercise, diet, and stress reduction.

HOW CANCER OCCURS

Sometimes cells are replaced in an uncontrolled way and may not have the organization required to function normally. They become unruly and display abnormal behavior by dividing too often and without order.

When this occurs, too much tissue develops. The tissue can be benign, as in the case of an enlarged prostate, or it can be cancerous. Because of their size, the growths or tumors move into adjacent areas and squeeze surrounding parts of the body. This will normally cause pain and interfere with body functions. These symptoms are rarely life-threatening, as we discussed in relation to BPH, but they are enough to get our attention.

If this excess tissue is noncancerous, we call it benign. The tumors that can spread to other parts of the body and that may be life-threatening we call malignant or cancerous. The body fluids that carry cancer cells are the blood and the lymph (a clear fluid that drains waste away from cells). These cells are found in many areas of the body, causing different types of cancer.

Prostate cancer usually starts with a tiny amount of cells that are located inside the prostate gland. They begin to divide and multiply abnormally. It usually takes slightly over one year for the tumor to double in size. Unfortunately, it cannot be detected at this stage by a digital rectal exam (DRE). It takes several more doublings before it can be felt by the doctor.

Most men will not notice any symptoms until the tumor reaches the size of a grape. As the tumor continues to grow, the symptoms common to BPH will occur, alerting the patient that something is going on down there.

Metastatic prostate cancer—that is, cancer that has spread beyond the prostate—follows a fairly predictable course. It first spreads to the lymph nodes, which lie next to the blood vessels that go to the legs, then it spreads along the channels that connect the lymph nodes. The malignant cells then enter the bones of the lower back. They spread to the upper back, ribs, and bones in the hips and legs. Pain is usually present. At this stage, the cancer has a large volume and can spread to the liver, lungs, and skin.

RISK FACTORS FOR PROSTATE CANCER

Many men can eat a high-fiber, low-fat diet, abstain from smoking, avoid the sun, and still develop prostate cancer. Other men do the opposite and do not develop prostate cancer. Why? There are many unknowns in the universe, and this is one of them.

We do know that eventually one in eleven men will get prostate cancer. We know that it generally occurs in middle-aged and elderly men, and that 80 percent of cases are diagnosed after age sixty-five. Many men die with prostate cancer without ever being aware that they had the disease. This is one of the major reasons there is an ongoing controversy as to whether treatment is always advisable.

Your odds of being afflicted with prostate cancer, based on age alone, are illustrated in the table below.

PROSTATE CANCER: WHAT ARE THE ODDS?

Current Age	Likelihood of Diagnosis This Year
40 to 44	1 in 58,824
45 to 49	1 in 13,158
50 to 54	1 in 2,667
55 to 59	1 in 874
60 to 64	1 in 348
65 to 69	1 in 174
70 to 74	1 in 115
75 to 79	1 in 90
80 to 84	1 in 80

As with other types of cancer, prostate cancer is easiest to treat when the tumor is confined to one spot, but 40 percent of prostate cancers are discovered after the disease has spread. The five-year survival rate for localized cancers is 85 percent; for all stages combined, 71 percent. Because it often has no symptoms, prostate cancer is commonly discovered too late for effective treatment.

According to Dr. Thomas Stamey, Professor of Urology at Stanford University School of Medicine, for every man who dies from cancer of the prostate, 380 more have microscopic evidence of cancer but do not die from it; most will die of heart disease and other causes. More than a million persons (primarily men) die of heart disease each year; forty million people suffer from diagnosed cardiovascular disease, and an even larger number don't know they have it. It's obvious, then, that a man with prostate cancer often will die of coronary problems before he succumbs to prostate cancer. Studies show that 30 percent of all American males have foci of adenocarcinoma (abnormal gland cells from the lining of an organ) of the prostate by age fifty; by age ninety, the incidence is 90 percent.

Genetic Causes

Doctors believe that some people have a genetic weakness that allows malignant cells to grow while others have a genetic resistance that seems to protect them regardless of how unhealthy their lifestyle may be. If only we could pick our ancestors, then we could diminish our chances of having cancer (needless to say, this option is not available to us).

Studies, as reviewed extensively in *Men's Confidential*, have shown that men whose male ancestors have had the disease are more at risk. If your father had prostate cancer, your risk is increased by two and a half times. If both your father and grandfather had this disease, your probability of getting it jumps by nine times.

Still, the explanation for this is not exactly clear. If both a father and son suffer from prostate cancer, is it because they were exposed to a dangerous environment or ate the same high-fat diet, or is it due to a genetic link?

In Iceland, Dr. Hiram Julius studied the possible genetic link of cancer among family members and came up with astonishing results. He calculated the rate of prostate cancer among relatives of 947 women who had breast cancer. Fathers, brothers, and sons of these women were roughly 1.4 times as likely to develop prostate cancer. Even second-degree relatives, such as uncles and nephews, were at about 1.2 times more risk. When nine women with breast cancer also had a first-degree relative with any of four types of cancer (breast, ovarian, endometrial, or prostate), her second-, third-, and even fourth-degree male relatives had 1.8 times the risk of developing prostate cancer.

The study makes one suspect that in Iceland the environment and lifestyle did not play as significant a role, as researchers investigated the medical histories of the husbands of the women with breast cancer and found increased risks in them as well. The new link between male and female cancers should put us on extra alert, and your doctor should be informed of your family history.

In the future, new research should be able to determine if your genetic makeup holds this risk factor for developing prostate cancer. Researchers have found a gene for early-onset prostate cancer, but not all prostate cancer. This gene appears to be implicated in the development of somewhat less than 10 percent of all cases of prostate cancer. However, it is responsible for almost one-half of the cases that occur in men who are fifty-five years of age or younger. The gene can be inherited from either the father or mother. Men who are at high risk of inheriting the gene are characterized by having a number of relatives who have a history of prostate cancer or a relative who had early-onset prostate cancer (stage A, as detailed later in this chapter).

Dr. Patrick C. Walsh, Chairman of Urology at Johns Hopkins University, has undertaken a massive study of families with a history of prostate cancer. He concludes that a man is at risk for hereditary prostate cancer if he meets any of the following criteria:

1. Three or more affected immediate family members (fathers, sons, brothers).
2. Three or more affected generations in either his maternal or paternal family lines.
3. Two immediate family members with early onset of prostate cancer (they became afflicted with the disease when they were younger than fifty-five years old).

If you fit this definition, Dr. Walsh advises that you begin screening for prostate cancer as early as age forty. The American Cancer Society echoes this advice.

According to a recent Montreal study, if a man has a brother who had prostate cancer, his chances of getting it are one in ten. When investigators studied the family histories of 6,000 men, they found that having a brother with prostate cancer made a man's chances of developing it two and a half times greater than for men without this family history and for men without prostate cancer.

The organization Patient Advocates for Advanced Cancer Treatments (PAACT) has accumulated data from over 8,000 patients, indicating the risk of getting prostate cancer based on family history:

History	Risk
No family history of cancer	1 in 9 (11.2 percent)
Family history of cancer other than prostate	2 in 9 (18.9 percent)
Both parents with cancer other than prostate	2 in 5 (42.6 percent)
Father had prostate cancer, mother other cancer	1 in 2 (53.1 percent)
Father and uncle had prostate cancer	3 in 5 (61.7 percent)
Grandfather, father, and uncles had prostate cancer	4 in 5 (86.3 percent)

These figures indicate that prostate cancer tends to be hereditary. If your father had prostate cancer and your mother had some form of cancer, there is a fifty-fifty chance that you will suffer from the disease. However, the probability that you will get prostate cancer increases depending on the number of family members on your father's side who had prostate cancer.

Location and Race

Where we are born, where we live, and what race we are may have a lot to do with our chances of being afflicted with prostate cancer. If you live in the United States or Western Europe, you have a greater risk of getting the disease than if you live in Asia or Eastern Europe.

According to Dr. Ruben F. Gittes, a physician with the Scripps Clinic Research Foundation in California, the incidence of clinically diagnosed prostatic cancer ranged from 0.8 cases per 100,000 males in Shanghai, China, to 100.1 per 100,000 among African-Americans living in Alameda County, California.

African-Americans have the highest prostate cancer risk worldwide and Caucasians have the second-highest risk; Japanese-Americans' risk rates are among the lowest. A recent survey by the California Department of Health Services found that African-Americans in California have a prostate cancer rate 37 percent higher than that of Caucasians, 100 percent higher than that of Latinos, and 217 percent higher than that of Asian-Americans.

Smoking

The role of smoking as a contributing factor to prostate cancer is being studied. Oral, throat, pancreas, lung, and bladder cancers are more common in smokers than in nonsmokers, and smoking is now recognized as contributing to prostate cancer.

If you are a smoker and you want to avoid getting prostate cancer, or you want to improve your chances of surviving this disease if it is already present, stop immediately. So advise researchers at the University of California at Davis Medical School, who studied

359 men with newly diagnosed prostate cancer. They found that the disease spreads earlier and more aggressively in smokers than in nonsmokers. Males who smoked more than one pack a day were twice as likely to develop advanced-stage prostate cancer as were nonsmokers or men who smoked less than half a pack a day.

As with lung cancer, if you stop smoking you have a good chance to stop the cancer from developing further. According to the *Journal of Radiology*, the use of tobacco products may mask cancer by inhibiting the changes in the PSA level and thereby not indicating the presence of cancer. This can disrupt the tracking process and delay the detection of prostate cancer until a later stage, when options to eliminate it are lessened. Researchers at the University of California at Davis Medical School reviewed records of 396 men under seventy-five years of age who had a history of transurethral prostatectomies and who had no prostate malignancy more advanced than stage A (see the "Stages of Prostate Cancer" section below). The data suggest smoking as a risk factor for stage A prostatic cancer and confirms smoking as a risk factor for prostatic hypertrophy requiring surgery.

Toxic Chemicals

Your yard may also be a danger to you if you use fertilizer or weed killers. Chemicals such as herbicides, fungicides, and insecticides should be eliminated from your life. One suggestion is to become an organic gardener. It may not only give you a better-looking yard, but it may help you to avoid prostate cancer as well. If you do use lawn chemicals, be sure that your body is completely covered. Wearing gloves, long sleeves, and pants to cover the skin is most important.

Researchers in North Carolina and Canada, after reviewing the census records of Canadian farmers over the age of 45, found a weak but significant correlation between the number of acres they sprayed with weed killer and their risk of death from prostate cancer.

Occupational Hazards

Studies of the effects of being employed in certain occupations have not been very convincing, but it appears that one way to stack the deck more in your favor in the fight against prostate cancer is to avoid occupations such as welding, sheet metal work, gardening, farming, janitorial work, working with cadmium in plating, or anything in the paper, rubber, or wood industries.

As happens so often in science, the data give rise to new questions. Are farmers, for example, at risk because they eat a diet that is higher in cholesterol or saturated fat? Or might the agricultural chemicals or longer exposure to the sun contribute to the farmers' susceptibility?

Sunshine

Some studies indicate a lower incidence of prostate cancer in areas of the world where people have greatest exposure to the sun. One researcher theorized that vitamin D, which is provided by the sun, acts as a cell regulator in the prostate; a lack of it may somehow lead to the development of prostate cancer.

Nonetheless, dermatologists will be quick to warn you that sun exposure can trigger melanoma, a type of skin cancer that is more deadly than prostate cancer.

Vasectomy

A study of 14,607 male nurses in eleven states suggested a link between vasectomies and prostate cancer. Dr. Edward Giovannucci correlated a 60 percent increase in the chances of the cancer in men who underwent the operation. Giovannucci observed that the risk was highest (89 percent) in men who had had a vasectomy over twenty years ago. In the first ten years after the vasectomy, there was no significant risk.

Many physicians see this matter differently however, notably Dr. Herbert Peterson, Chief of the Women's Health and Fertility Branch of the Centers for Disease Control and Prevention in Atlanta. "The association between vasectomy and prostate cancer is not strong; there are two other good studies that found no link, and there is no known biological explanation for a link. It does not make sense," Dr. Peterson said. He pointed out that the majority of men who develop prostate cancer have not undergone a vasectomy. "We spent a whole decade on a wild goose chase exploring the link between vasectomy and heart disease," Dr. Peterson said. "We consistently see that men with vasectomies are healthier and live longer. This is a puzzle that will take some time to resolve."

Patients who have had a vasectomy can be further reassured by an American Urological Association task force that criticized two recent studies linking vasectomy to prostate cancer. They concluded that the studies were scientifically flawed, and resolved that men who have had vasectomies do not need to be tested more frequently than usual for prostate cancer. The task force also pointed out that new information has become available this spring that shows these men are not at increased risk.

Researchers from several major universities also conducted a vasectomy study of over 3,000 newly diagnosed prostate cancer patients and control subjects, including African-Americans, Caucasians, Chinese-Americans, and Japanese-Americans (subjects in past studies were mostly Caucasian). Dr. Esther M. John, an epidemiologist at the Northern California Center and lead researcher of the vasectomy study, said, "We did not find any statistically significant association between vasectomies and cancer…. That conclusion applied regardless of ethnicity. We can't say why other studies found an association and we didn't; I don't think this question is completely resolved yet."

"Vasectomy has become one of the most accepted forms of contraception in this country, and this study finds it does not increase the risk of prostate cancer. While nothing is ever permanent, men should take a lot of solace from this finding," agreed Dr. Ralph W. deVere White, chairman of the Department of Urology at the University of California at Davis Medical Center.

HOW PROSTATE CANCER DEVELOPS

Prostate cancer, like other forms of cancer, begins as a tiny change in just a few cells. Prostate cancer usually grows very slowly over the first several years. But, sooner or later, it will grow at a much faster rate and can become fatal. Detecting it early will not only catch it before it spreads but will also call for a less extreme method of treatment.

Physicians have many tools available to determine the size and the stage, or extent of the spread, of prostate cancer. Many use the older ABCD system, while others classify prostate cancer by the TNM (tumor, nodes, metastases) system. Each classification has subdivisions, which are described below.

Stages of Prostate Cancer

Staging is a system used by doctors to determine the extent of the cancer and how to treat it. By understanding the stages of cancer, a patient can, with his doctor, make fully informed decisions regarding treatment. Unfortunately, as discussed earlier, symptoms are not always apparent to alert us.

Stage A In stage A, a doctor cannot feel a tumor during the digital rectal exam (DRE), and the patient has no symptoms. The cancer is typically discovered when portions of the prostate are removed to treat BPH; during the subsequent biopsy, microscopic areas of cancer are found. If the biopsy indicates that the cancer that is present is not more than 5 percent of the tissue, then it is considered to be in substage A1. A cancer with more than this percentage is in substage A2. Depending on the health, age, and decision of the patient, a radical prostatectomy (removal of the prostate gland and surrounding tissues) will often be recommended.

Stage B In stage B, the cancer is confined to the prostate gland. At this stage, the patient may not notice symptoms to alert him to the problem. The doctor may detect its presence during the DRE, and the level of PSA may be increased. As with stage A, stage B is divided into substages. If the tumor is detected in only one lobe of the prostate and is about two centimeters (three-quarters of an inch) in diameter, it is classified as stage B1. If it is in more than one lobe, or it is greater than two centimeters, it is classified as B2. Surgery or radiation hormone therapy may be an option if the patient is older and is not considered in good enough health for surgery.

Stage C In stage C, the cancer cells have spread outside the capsule, or covering, of the prostate gland into tissues around the prostate. The symptoms indicate something is not right down there. The spread may reach the glands that produce semen. Unfortunately, most patients don't visit their doctor until this stage, when the doctor may have to resort to radiation therapy.

Stage D In stage D, the cancer has spread outside the prostate capsule and has invaded the lymph nodes, bone marrow, lungs, liver, or other parts of the body. If the cancer has progressed to lymph nodes in the pelvic area, it is classified as D1. In D2, it has spread to remote parts of the body. There is often considerable pain, especially in the upper thigh, lower back, and pelvic area. If the cancer has spread to the bones or lymph nodes, there is no known cure. The doctor will try to control the disease by eliminating the male hormones, which stimulate the growth and spread of the cancer.

The TNM System

The TNM system is being used more by physicians, not only in the United States but in other countries as well. The letter T (tumor) describes the cancer with different numbers to indicate the size of the cancer. N (nodes) tells us if the cancer has spread to the lymph nodes; N1, N2, and N3 relate to the size and number of nodes involved. M (metastases) indicates if the cancer has spread to distant lymph nodes or to remote areas such as the bones, liver, or lungs.

CHAPTER FOUR

Diagnosing Prostate Problems

Men who develop prostate problems may be tempted to end their relationship with their prostate gland immediately. One way to do that is to have the testicles removed, so the circulating hormone that contributes to the enlarging of the prostate ceases to flow. But that, needless to say, would not be a popular choice. Besides, by the time the prostate starts to cause problems, it has probably reached its maximum size.

Another option is to remove the prostate surgically. This choice can be very tempting as the symptoms become increasingly annoying. After all, if the gland is removed, no essential function is impaired—if, that is, you no longer want to father a child.

There are several periods in your life when you might seriously consider parting company with your prostate because of the problems it causes you (and there is no shortage of urologists ready to accommodate you). These periods can be divided into age groups. In the first period (ages twenty-five to forty), an inflammation of the prostate may give you a wake-up call to say "Here I am," and the term prostate is added to your vocabulary. In the second period (ages forty-five to fifty), your prostate gland may reintroduce itself by developing BPH. In the third period (around age fifty), prostate cancer may occur.

DETECTION AND DIAGNOSIS

To live a long and healthy life, you should schedule an annual physical examination once you reach the age of forty. The American Cancer Society recommends that every man over forty years of age have a digital rectal examination (DRE) as part of his annual physical checkup—although less than 25 percent do so. It also recommends that men over fifty years of age have an annual prostate-specific antigen (PSA) blood test; men who are at high risk for prostate cancer (see Chapter 3) should begin getting both the DRE and the PSA blood test before the age of fifty. If the results of either the DRE or PSA blood test are suspicious, a transrectal ultrasound (TRUS) and biopsy normally follow.

Some men adopt a wait-and-see attitude: they will go with the roll of the dice, and if it happens, it happens. But a more sensible attitude is this: if it is going to happen, you want to know about it as soon as it occurs to improve your odds of surviving.

It has been estimated that between the years 1990 and 2000 the number of cases of prostate cancer will increase by 90 percent, and that deaths from prostate cancer will increase by 37 percent. (The figures in 1996 are already surpassing that estimate.) These figures are assuming that no new means of detection and treatment are developed. The numbers are grim, but they are an important incentive for men to go in for that prostate exam.

THE EXAMINATION

Before going for your checkup, it is helpful to the physician if you jot down information relevant to your health. Many doctors agree that a well-taken history can be as important as the examination. Former laboratory results should be gathered as well as any other medical records that you have compiled over the years.

You should share intimate details with your doctor pertaining to family matters. Problems at home or at the workplace can have a definite impact on your overall health. Ideally, the doctor will be a good listener and treat you, the patient, rather than the disease.

Urine Testing

As part of the examination, a urine sample will be taken. Urinalysis can tell the doctor a great deal about you, and it is helpful in detecting mild inflammations as well as serious tumors. It can alert the doctor to look further for what may be a serious disorder. If infection in the urinary tract is to be properly diagnosed, a culture of the urine is necessary. It is an important tool to also detect disorders of the kidney, bladder, and liver, including malignant cells in these vital organs.

The Digital Rectal Examination (DRE)

Most doctors consider the DRE to be the easiest, least expensive, and most useful method of diagnosing and analyzing diseases of the prostate, especially in their earliest and most curable stages. If your doctor does not give you a DRE during your physical exam, you should demand that it be done. DREs have been in use for many years, and they were the only screening tool for prostate cancer until TRUS and PSA tests became widely available in the 1980s.

The DRE is brief and involves little discomfort. The doctor performs the exam by inserting a lubricated, gloved finger into the patient's rectum to feel the size and shape of the prostate gland, which is located adjacent to the rectum and about an inch from the anal opening. An enlarged gland could indicate cancer, but it is more often a result of BPH. If the prostate is normal, it will have a smooth surface. A malignant tumor, however, may be felt as a small, hard nodule. If a tumor grows, this nodule will enlarge and more nodules may appear.

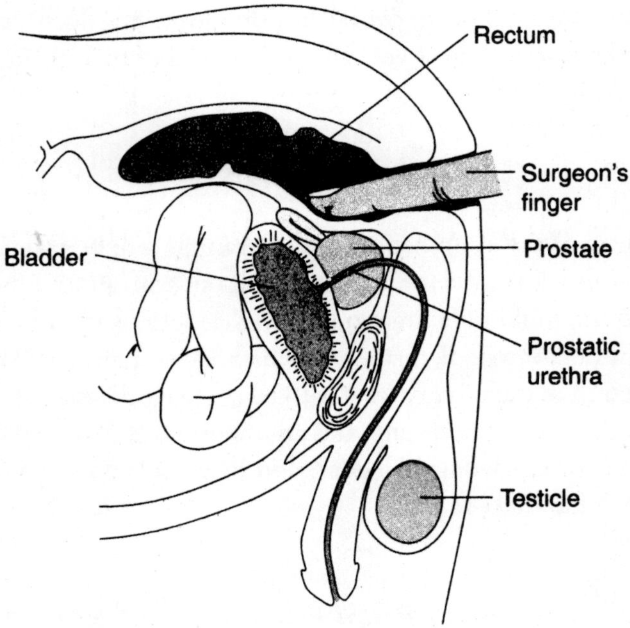

THE DIGITAL RECTAL EXAM

Far too many doctors do not perform this procedure. The infrequency in which it is performed is inexcusable. The U.S. Department of Health and Human Services has estimated that only one out of ten men in the appropriate age group receive an annual rectal exam. From 1989 to 1990, the Cleveland Clinic studied 433 men over the age of forty. It determined that 67 percent of the men had not had a DRE performed in the previous year. More bad news was that although 153 men did have a general physical examination in the previous year, the DRE was included only about 56 percent of the time.

This widespread neglect sets men up for enduring a long and painful disease; 50 percent of cancerous tissue is discovered after it has spread, when it is too late to effectively treat it.

As important as the DRE is, it is not infallible. Less than 20 percent of prostate cancers can be detected by the DRE. Some cancers are too small to be felt, and cancerous growths that are located in the front part of the prostate gland cannot be reached in the DRE. Malignant cells that do not form a distinct, touchable nodule may also escape detection.

The Prostate-Specific Antigen (PSA) Test

Most physicians will also order the PSA test. When the DRE is performed in conjunction with the PSA test, the detection rate for prostate cancer increases significantly, to between 53 and 70 percent. Based on an antigen (a class of substances produced by the body that stimulates production of antibodies) discovered in 1971, the PSA has recently attracted a lot of media attention. Many doctors consider it to be a promising test for detecting prostate cancer.

The prostate-specific antigen is produced naturally in the prostate gland and nowhere else in the body. As the prostate enlarges, it may cause slightly higher levels of this antigen in the blood, because there is more of the prostate to produce more antigen. When cancerous cells are present in the prostate, they spread to other parts of the body and then also produce PSA. Since malignant prostate tissue makes considerably more of the antigen than normal tissue, the test alerts the physician to possible malignant cell activity.

A major problem with the PSA test is that it does not distinguish between prostate cancer that will not pose a serious problem (given a man's life expectancy at the time of diagnosis) and a dangerous type that may invade the bone. This results in a tough call for both the patient and the surgeon. In fact, Norman Yang, one of the scientists who identified the PSA, commented recently that he has serious doubts about the value of his discovery. Nevertheless, most urologists regard the PSA test as an important tool in diagnosing prostate cancer.

Many physicians recommend that a patient not have a PSA test taken after a DRE, as there is some concern that it would affect the measurement. However, an extensive study reported in the *Journal of the American Medical Association (JAMA)* concluded that no clinically important effects on serum PSA levels were noticed after a DRE.

The cost for a PSA test is approximately $50. It will take from twenty-four to seventy-two hours to receive the results. The PSA test results are not affected by when you eat; they may be influenced by ejaculation, but probably not significantly.

Many doctors use the following figures as a guide to normal PSA levels for various age groups:

Age	Normal PSA Level Range
40 to 49	0 to 2.5 ng/ml*
50 to 59	0 to 3.5 ng/ml
60 to 69	0 to 4.5 ng/ml
70 to 79	0 to 6.5 ng/ml

*ng/ml: nanograms per milliliter of blood

There are doctors who feel that these figures are not appropriate for screening. According to a study reported at the 1993 American Urological Association meeting, an annual increase in PSA levels of about 0.04 ng/ml is not abnormal as men's age and size increases, especially over the age of sixty. Several benign conditions, including BPH, prostatitis, and prostatic blockage, can elevate the serum PSA level. As a result, approximately 20 percent of patients without clinically evident prostate cancer will have elevated PSA levels.

It is also important to realize that a normal PSA level does not mean that you do not have cancer. The cancer may be too small or too primitive to produce much PSA.

If you do have a PSA level above the normal range for your age, your doctor may perform a biopsy, which involves taking a sample of tissue to be analyzed under a microscope. You will probably also be referred to a urologist.

The Urological Examination

A urologist is a doctor who has had extensive training in the physiology and pathology of the genitourinary tract. This training usually lasts for five or six years after medical school. The doctor then must pass a day-long written examination given by the Board of Urology. After a year and a half, if the doctor's practice of urology is considered competent, he or she must then demonstrate satisfactory expertise before a committee in an orals examination before becoming board-certified and receiving the title of Diplomate of the American Board of Urology—a prestigious and highly coveted designation. The considerable training and experience of a board-certified urologist should give you a high level of confidence.

Men are typically apprehensive about a urological exam; there is a special fear about having a doctor examine what's between their legs. But—to put it literally—you are in the hands of an expert. The exam is usually without pain, and the results will often give you peace of mind. The urologist will most likely begin by feeling the patient's lower abdomen to see if the bladder is full. One of the common developments associated with BPH is residual urine, which can build up to such a volume that the bladder becomes distended.

A urine sample will be taken once more; again, this is basically a screening test to provide pertinent information about a patient and his genitourinary tract at a bargain cost. The urologist will look for red blood cells in the urine, which suggest disease in the urinary tract, BPH, bladder infection, bladder cancer, bladder or kidney stones, kidney cancer, or prostate cancer. If red blood cells are present, an X-ray of the urethra and bladder may be recommended. White blood cells (pus cells) in the urine could also alert the doctor to an infection. Although examining the urine sample does not directly contribute to the diagnosis of BPH or prostate cancer, the analysis is a basic and valuable tool for the urologist and well worth the cost.

The patient may also undergo a urodynamic study—a test with a flow meter to determine the flow rate of the urine. This will help the doctor determine whether the patient's symptoms are the result of an obstruction or a different problem, such as bladder abnormalities. In some cases, the doctor will elect to use a catheter to measure the urine left in the bladder after urinating (alternatively, this can now be done more comfortably using a small ultrasound machine).

The PSA test and the DRE will most likely be given again. The urologist may very well detect a problem that was overlooked by a family physician not experienced in giving a DRE. If the patient was referred to the urologist, he or she will certainly want to establish whether or not a problem may exist. The urologist will also want another PSA test, as often a result will vary, and they will want to ascertain a reliable level for future testing.

A variety of sophisticated equipment is available for diagnosing prostate problems. The urologist will order the tests necessary to make an accurate diagnosis. You should discuss these options at length with your urologist; you will feel more relaxed about subjecting yourself to these procedures if you understand why they are ordered. Following are some of the available options.

CT or CAT Scan

CAT stands for computerized axial tomography (that name alone ought to strike fear in any malignant cells!). The CAT scan combines the use of X-ray and computer technology. Its major use is to determine the nature of tissues and whether a tissue mass is benign or if it is dense enough to be a malignant tumor.

The CAT scan machine revolves around a patient's body and takes a series of X-rays. A computer interprets this information by converting the X-rays into photographic images and creating detailed views of the tissues of the body. The results are more revealing than standard X-rays. The procedure is painless and takes about an hour.

A CAT scan involves more radiation than does a chest X-ray, but the patient will not be exposed to a significant amount as long as he is not undergoing the procedure frequently. The CAT scan is not considered 100 percent accurate, but it can be helpful in evaluating the progress of a tumor. However, it is not required in 90 percent of patients with prostate cancer. A major limitation of the CAT scan is in its assessment of lymph nodes, small masses of tissue that remove bacteria and other toxins from the body. The nodes must be visibly abnormal in order to arouse suspicion. Thus, lymph nodes with microscopic metastasis (spread of malignant cells to another part of the body) often will not be detected. At other times, the nodes can look enlarged and very suspicious, yet the pathologist (a doctor who specializes in the examination of cells and tissues that are removed from the body) will find no evidence of cancer.

Bone Scan

A bone scan employs a nuclear-medicine body imaging technique in which a tiny amount of radioactive substance is injected into the bloodstream. When cancer spreads, it often spreads to the bone. When the bone is damaged, new bone is produced by the body's natural healing process. The bone scan can detect such a repair, alerting the urologist that cancer may have spread to the bone.

This diagnostic tool is considered by many urologists to be one of the most sensitive imaging techniques for identifying cancer in the bone. A very low dose of a radioactive substance is injected into the body, and it then filters its way into the skeletal structure and collects in areas where bone repair has occurred. After the substance is injected, there is a one-hour wait; the scanning process then takes about thirty minutes. The bone scan is painless and can be performed at an outpatient clinic. The main drawback of this test is that if the patient has other problems such as arthritis, an infection, or a fracture, the bone scan cannot distinguish that damage from cancer damage.

As a side note, it is interesting that researchers have discovered the likely reason why prostate cancer so often spreads into the backbone: the bone tissue is rich in a protein that sharply stimulates the growth of prostate tumor cells. The new work suggests that advanced prostate cancer may be amenable to treatment by blocking the activity of the stimulatory protein, a molecule called transferrin.

Magnetic Resonance Imaging (MRI)

Many urologists find MRI to be the most useful imaging tool around. It creates high-quality pictures of the internal organs far sharper than those produced by a CAT scan. MRI involves using an electromagnet to stimulate the hydrogen molecules in the water in the body. As these molecules vibrate, they give off small electrical charges that are sensed by the MRI machine and translated into an image. No radiation is involved, as MRI makes use of a magnetic field and radio-frequency signals.

MRI presents superior pictures, and it is a precise tool for viewing the internal makeup of the brain, spinal cord, and bones. It is normally used by doctors not to diagnose prostate cancer but rather to see what stage it is in so they can best decide how to treat it. Aside from surgery, it is the most sensitive test for observing the spread of the disease through the prostate capsule or seminal vesicles.

A newer use for the MRI is in early detection, through the use of small probes that have been developed for the transrectal MRI, which are placed in the rectum. Some urologists believe this is helpful in preventing unnecessary biopsies, although others question the procedure. If costs come down, it may be used more for the detection of prostate cancer in the early stage.

The MRI tells the doctor if abnormalities in the bones are due to cancer, but it does not provide any additional information about the lymph nodes, which are a common site for the spread of malignant cells.

The MRI causes no pain and can be done in about thirty minutes on an outpatient basis. It only hurts in the pocketbook, but it is covered by insurance and Medicare. When you get your bill for this procedure, keep in mind that the cost of the machine is in the millions.

Ultrasound

Ultrasound involves no radiation exposure and practically no risk. Since there is also very little pain or discomfort, patients are usually very receptive to this technique.

Prostate ultrasonography is a method of determining prostate volume, which, in relation to the level of serum PSA, is a guide to the likelihood of the presence of cancer. Sonographic guidance can enhance the accuracy of prostatic biopsy (see below), particularly of small lesions.

Ultrasound is similar to the sonar used by the Navy during World War II to detect enemy submarines beneath the surface of the ocean. In the ultrasound procedure, a series of high-frequency sound waves are generated by a probe that is inserted in the rectum. The sound waves that bounce off of human tissues are transmitted as electrical signals to a screen that presents a picture of—in this case—the entire prostate. During the ultrasound exam, the doctor can point out on the screen what is going on, which is very interesting and reassuring to the patient. The images can also be recorded.

Ultrasound is helpful to a doctor in determining the size of the gland so that the best surgical approach can be used. It is best at "seeing" solid organs in the abdomen and soft tissues wherever the signal won't be stopped by intervening bone or air; it's not very useful in the chest, bowel, or head. Sound travels well through liquids, which means that ultrasound is very good at distinguishing solid tumors from fluid-filled cysts.

Many urologists use a transrectal technique, in which an ultrasound probe covered with a rubber balloon is filled with water (to provide the liquid medium for the ultrasound) and placed into the rectum with very little pain. This provides an ultrasonic picture of the prostate and the bladder. Some doctors feel that the procedure is more helpful in discovering cancers that have spread beyond the prostate than in detecting very early ones. But others say that it can also aid them in diagnosing a very small prostate cancer.

One advantage of transrectal ultrasonography is that when the apparatus is in the rectum, in addition to producing sound waves it can guide needles to remove some tissue from the prostate for a biopsy (see below).

Ultrasound is not perfect, but it is another tool that is helpful in indicating what type of treatment should be used on a patient. It can be performed either in a doctor's office or at a hospital.

Some researchers have found that the ultrasound exam did a poor job of predicting which areas of the prostate to biopsy. Areas that looked suspicious on the ultrasound were not necessarily found to be cancerous during biopsy, and areas that looked normal sometimes did harbor cancer. According to one study, biopsying only areas that looked suspicious on ultrasound would have caused 24.6 percent of patients with prostate cancer to be missed.

Intravenous Prelogram (IVP)

For this form of X-ray, a dye is injected into the forearm of the patient. The dye is filtered out of the blood by the kidneys, at which point the X-ray can provide considerable information about the bladder, the kidneys, and the entire urinary tract. Kidney stones, obstruction by scars, or cancer may be detected. It can also point out whether the cancer has spread. The exam takes about an hour and can be done in the doctor's office.

Cystoscopy

Cystoscopy is a very brief procedure used when blood is observed in the urine or to detect bladder cancers. It involves the use of a hollow instrument that looks like a skinny periscope, or, in many cases, a flexible tube containing two very thin tubes. The first tube is used to insert fluid into the area being observed. The second tube contains a light and lenses so that the physician is able to see into the bladder and urethra with great accuracy. The instrument is inserted into the urethral opening at the end of the penis and slowly advanced into the bladder. Most urologists will only use cystoscopy if they have reason to suspect a bladder tumor stone or other irregular condition; it is not used routinely to detect prostate problems. The procedure is not very painful and can be performed in a doctor's office.

Biopsy

If the results of a test look suspicious, the urologist will probably want to perform a biopsy. Biopsy is a frightening word for most people.

The prostatic biopsy is a minor surgical procedure that can be done either in a doctor's office or in a hospital; the patient should be able to play golf or tennis the next day. A special needle is inserted through the rectum, and a small piece of tissue is obtained from the targeted area. The procedure takes about ten minutes, and the patient feels only slight discomfort, similar to an injection; a local anesthetic can be used, although often no anesthesia is used at all. A high-speed "biopsy gun" uses a smaller needle, takes just a few thousandths of a second, and causes less pain.

Biopsy results are usually available within forty-eight hours. The pathologist examines the tissues under a microscope for signs of malignant cells. Typically, several pathologists will look at a sample to ensure agreement on the diagnosis, so mistakes are considered rare.

Another biopsy method is the "tru cut" biopsy, in which a large hollow needle is used to remove a core or plug of prostate tissue, which is then examined under the microscope. This is a more painful procedure, with an increased risk of infection. Many physicians feel that a minimum of six punctures should be performed during this procedure and that it should be undertaken in conjunction with a transrectal ultrasound examination.

SECOND THOUGHTS ON PSA TESTS

The routine use of the PSA test is questioned on five counts:

1. It has not been used over a long enough period of time to establish its accuracy.
2. Treating the cancers it discovers may not save lives.
3. The cost of screening all men over the age of fifty would be high.
4. About 42 percent of men with early organ-confined prostate cancers (the ones most likely to benefit from early detection) do not have elevated PSA levels.
5. A high rate of false positive results can lead to unnecessary biopsies in about four out of ten cases (consequently, many health plans are reluctant to finance PSAs).

Research performed in the Department of Radiology at St. Joseph Mercy Hospital in Ann Arbor, Michigan, showed that "as males age, there is a growth of benign glandular tissue that causes an elevation of PSA. The danger of what is happening today is that many men with a high PSA are worried that they have prostate cancer unnecessarily. Therefore, when the PSA is elevated, the next step is to correlate with the size of the gland." The prostate can vary in size from that of a pea to that of an apple; as the prostate enlarges, the PSA level also increases.

Proponents of the PSA test say that it may not be perfect, but at the present time it is the best tool we have. Under the screening strategy, a biopsy is performed when a nodule is found by a DRE or when the PSA value is greater than 10 ng/ml. When the DRE is negative and the PSA is 4 ng/ml to 10 ng/ml, the PSA density (the PSA level divided by the prostate volume) is used to determine the need for a biopsy.

PSAs and Biopsies

Urologists such as Dr. Fred Lee, a clinical professor in radiology and urology at Wayne State University in Detroit, express alarm about the increase in the number of biopsies as a result of using the PSA as a screening test. While Dr. Lee agrees with the practice of recommending a biopsy to men with PSA blood levels higher than 10 ng/ml, he takes issue with the common practice of ordering ultrasound and an immediate biopsy for men who fall within the gray area between 4 ng/ml and 10 ng/ml (a large portion of the older male population who have BPH are within this range).

According to Dr. Lee, a biopsy, "which is often presented as a harmless approach, does pose a risk to the patient. Because the biopsy sample is taken through the rectum, the process introduces bacteria into the prostate. Although prophylactic antibiotics are given, they don't reach high levels in the prostate.

"[The prostate is] a gland that doesn't concentrate antibiotics very well. Once a man gets a low-grade infection in the prostate, it tends to stay for a long time. Then the PSA goes higher, the patient goes in for another checkup, and what does the doctor do? He biopsies a second time. So they're in a vicious cycle."

A new development in PSA testing may prevent unnecessary biopsies for the 25 percent of men with PSA levels in the 4 ng/ml to 10 ng/ml range. The PSA test spots two kinds of molecules: free and complexed. The latter are associated with cancer and are difficult to spot, whereas the free molecules are easy to spot and are associated with an enlarged prostate or recent ejaculation. When investigators studied the ratio of free to total PSA in 115 men with total levels ranging from 4 ng/ml to 10 ng/ml, they discovered that a ratio greater than 1.5 accurately indicated an absence of cancer. They suggested using this ratio to lower the number of men getting biopsies. A new national trial involving 12,000 patients at eight medical centers around the U.S. has been launched in an effort to verify results.

PSAs and Watchful Waiting

The main flaw of the PSA test has been that a high reading may only indicate enlargement of the prostate due to infection or irritation and not cancer, thus leading to unnecessary surgery. A study by a team at Johns Hopkins University resulted in a process for fine-tuning the PSA test to solve this problem. In this study, each man's PSA density was calculated, then the men's prostates were biopsied to allow microscopic evaluation of tissue. Six cores of tissue from various sections of the prostate were removed. The Hopkins researchers estimated that tumors would be nonaggressive in 11 percent of the men with PSA levels over 4 ng/ml. Subsequent surgical examination of all of the men's prostates proved that this prediction was correct.

As a result, new guidelines were established for watchful waiting, also called deferred maintenance or active surveillance. In this process, the doctor monitors the patient on a regular schedule, as long as patients fulfill the following criteria:

- Their PSA density must be less than 0.15 (a PSA value that is 15 percent of the total weight of the prostate gland, as estimated by ultrasound).
- No more than two cores of prostate tissue removed at biopsy should show any evidence of cancer.

- Less than 50 percent of any single biopsy core should contain cancer cells.
- Any cancer cells must be "less aggressive," meaning that they are likely to be slow growing.

Additionally, a patient's age is taken into account. Because prostate cancer is slow growing, older men with small tumors can more safely opt for watchful waiting than can younger men. Men in their fifties and early sixties who have prostate cancer are likely to live long enough for their disease to develop, while men in their late seventies and eighties are likely to die from something else before their prostate tumors can become life-threatening. "Men in their upper sixties with insignificant tumors are particularly good candidates for watchful waiting," according to Dr. Patrick C. Walsh of the Johns Hopkins Medical Institution in Baltimore.

Other Considerations

Another important consideration in screening was revealed by a recent study undertaken at the Mayo Clinic comparing the physiology of Japanese and Caucasian men. Because of physiological differences, particularly the size of the prostate gland, the normal levels of PSA differed between the two races. Japanese men tend to have smaller prostates; therefore, a PSA level that is considered normal for a Caucasian man may indicate the presence of cancer in a Japanese man.

Dr. Joseph E. Oesterling, Chief Urologist at the Michigan Medical Center in Ann Arbor, comments that more research is needed to further outline the racial differences in PSA norms, especially among African-American men, who have a higher risk of prostate cancer.

Another important consideration concerns men who use the drug Finasteride (Proscar). This drug is used by many males to treat problems of BPH. It works by lowering the level of male hormones within the prostate gland, in which case the PSA level could go down as much as 50 percent. These levels could be very misleading; many doctors question the value of PSA testing with men who are using Finasteride.

PSA Tests: An Overview

An article in *Cancer Journal* provides an overview of this clinical dilemma in screening for prostate cancer. It states that any current diagnostic test can decrease mortality, but new information about optimal combinations of DRE, transrectal ultrasound, and the PSA test suggest that their combined predictive values can identify not only men at high risk but also those for whom continued frequent screening may not be cost-effective.

According to Dr. Ralph W. deVere White and associates from the University of California at Davis, PSA levels obtained from urine can be as accurate as those from blood. The team evaluated forty-three patients following radical prostatectomies and found that 77 percent of the patients had elevated urinary PSA, while only 33 percent had elevated serum (blood) PSA levels. They concluded that following surgery, close to 80 percent of the patients had tumor-bearing prostate tissues remaining locally, which the standard PSA blood tests did not recognize.

Overall, the study revealed that most men's urinary PSA level matched the blood serum PSA level, except following surgery. The investigators noted that after radical prostatectomies, urine PSA elevations were twice as common as elevated blood serum PSA levels. This suggested to the team that more patients have residual cancer than has previously been suspected.

The investigators will have to do more research before they are ready to claim that postoperative clinical treatment will be required for men whose urine PSA level is elevated while their blood serum PSA level is not.

Despite the shortcomings of the PSA test, the American Cancer Society and the American Urological Association recommend annual PSA testing for men beginning at age fifty, or at age forty if their family history puts them at a high risk for cancer. "Better to overdiagnose than underdiagnose," says cancer researcher Curtis Mettlin, "because by the time we find 40 percent of these cancers, it's too late to cure them."

Bob Dole, whose cancer was detected with the PSA test, encourages others to be tested. "I'm one of the many men who consider themselves living proof that early detection can mean a healthy future. Please have routine checkups, and don't neglect to have your doctor check for prostate disease. It could save your life."

It is interesting to note the attitudes of Europeans regarding diagnostic tests for prostate cancer. In northern Europe, PSA and DRE tests are not routinely used. Doctors there are concerned that indiscriminate use of these tests will lead to overdiagnosis and overtreatment. Information on the effectiveness of treatment from randomized trials is unavailable, and no evidence exists that early diagnosis and treatment will lead to an improvement of disease-related and overall mortality.

PSA vs. Quality of Life A new study adds more fuel to the debate. A *JAMA* report concluded that screening all men for prostate cancer is not cost-effective and doesn't significantly extend life. Based on the analysis, screening all men once, using the PSA test and a DRE, would add only six days to the life expectancies of fifty-year-old men and 1.7 days for seventy-year-old men. However, critics say that the report was based on statistics and assumptions and not clinical data.

Dr. Gerald Chodak, Professor of Surgery at the University of Chicago, is a vocal critic of the American Cancer Society's recommendations regarding PSA testing. "What I am for is providing better information to patients," he told *Modern Medicine*. "We don't know that screening will lower mortality from prostate cancer.

Until we do, the ACS shouldn't be making recommendations, and we should not be telling patients that screening will save their lives."

This argument doesn't make sense to Dr. Gerald P. Murphy, former Chief Medical Officer at the American Cancer Society. "We're not finding cancers that don't need treatment," he says. In one study of men who were diagnosed with prostate cancer by PSA and DRE, 85 percent of the cancers found were clinically significant.

PSAs, DREs, and Early Screenings A study that speaks highly of the PSA when performed in conjunction with a DRE was cited by Dr. E. David Crawford at the University of Colorado Health Sciences Center in Denver. He presented results obtained from 25,954 men who had prostate exams. Among a subgroup of 4,035 patients who had follow-up biopsies, 41.6 percent of those with elevated levels of PSA were found to have proscate cancer. Of the patients who had abnormal DREs, only 20 percent had prostate cancer. A positive predictive value of 44 percent was found when both tests were used.

"If you believe that screening is a worthwhile endeavor, then the combination of the two tests is better than either one alone," he told *Modern Medicine*. These data confirm the results of a 1991 study conducted by researchers at Washington University School of Medicine in St. Louis, Missouri, which concluded that the PSA test appears to be reliable. The researchers also determined that the combination of PSA testing and rectal examination with ultrasonography performed in patients with abnormal findings provides a better method of detecting prostate cancer than rectal examinations alone.

The PSA test is beneficial for early screening of cancer, according to a more recent study conducted by Dr. Charles Hennekens of Harvard Medical School and Brigham and Women's Hospital in Boston. It involved data from a continuing research project that included 22,071 doctors who were forty-two to eighty-four years old in 1982.

A survey to estimate the incidence of prostate cancer in Olmsted County, Minnesota, from 1983 through 1992 concluded that the increase is due in part to the expanded utilization of PSA testing; the more testing that is done, the more cancer will be found. The study also suggested that in terms of making a diagnosis, early detection efforts may be effective in identifying more early-stage, smaller cancers.

The PSA test can be valuable for patients who have prostate cancer and want to adopt a wait-and-see approach rather than go right into surgery. "A doctor who discovers a patient has prostate cancer must always ask the question, 'How big is the cancer?' As long as it's less than a milliliter in volume—about the size of a sugar cube—the patient doesn't need any therapy. He is far more likely to die of something else long before the prostate cancer spreads enough to bother him," said Dr. Thomas Stamey. To keep tabs on a tumor, doctors should monitor the patient with an annual PSA blood test, Stamey said. If the tumor grows larger, the patient may be a candidate for surgery.

The PSA test is also a good way to monitor the progress of prostate cancers after surgery or radiation treatment. Dr. Anthony Zietman, a radiation oncologist at Massachusetts General Hospital (MGH), recently completed a study that affirmed the value of PSA tests in determining the most appropriate course of treatment and in predicting the likelihood of patients remaining cancer-free. Study results indicate that understanding the significance of specific PSA levels prior to treatment can help determine which patients will do well with radiation therapy alone and which patients will benefit from more aggressive treatment combining radiation therapy, surgery, and endocrine therapy. Establishing a baseline PSA level is important so it can be monitored to see how it is affected by a form of treatment.

Though PSA testing has been used routinely as a follow-up tool after prostate cancer treatment, the results of the MGH study indicate that by lowering what is considered an acceptable level of

PSA, a recurrence of cancer can be detected earlier, allowing further treatment to begin at a more beneficial stage.

It is still undetermined whether the PSA test given yearly will reduce the death rate. The National Cancer Institute recently began a trial of 37,000 men, which will help to answer that question in ten years.

During the tracking stage, it is important to remember that there are actually two types of PSA: complexed and free. Since different tests will weigh the two types in a dissimilar manner, the results reported by different labs can be confusing to a patient. Fortunately, this is about to change. An international group of researchers, clinicians, and pharmaceutical executives from around the world met recently and agreed to use a common standard for reporting PSA test results.

PART II

What to Do If You Have BPH

CHAPTER FIVE

Watchful Waiting

If you develop an enlarged prostate, you will not be alone. If everyone discussed it openly, you might be amazed at how many of your associates share the same problem. Having company is not enough, however; you need a strategy for monitoring the condition of your prostate. The symptoms of an enlarged prostate are similar to those of prostate cancer. How will you know which you have? And how will you decide whether to treat the condition or when or how to treat it?

The better a patient understands his condition, the better his chances are of making the right choices. It is important to become aware of the pros and cons of various tests and options. Most important is that you have a doctor with whom you can communicate. It is advisable to include your mate, if you have one, in discussions about your condition and your options.

Remember that it may be better to be treated now than later, when a change in your overall physical condition may diminish the chances of success. If a prostate problem is caught at an early stage, the odds are greatly in your favor that you will make it through this ordeal and the quality of your life will be restored.

On the other hand, after reviewing the literature and talking with your doctor in depth, you may decide to wait a while longer. There are no simple ways to determine the best course to follow; the choice will depend on your health and other factors. The fear of complications from surgery or another treatment is also a major factor when thinking about waiting (show me the man who doesn't panic at the thought of a doctor moving a knife around between his legs!).

A VIABLE OPTION

Many men do elect to watch and wait. A patient's symptoms will determine to a great extent if he is a successful candidate for the option of watchful waiting. If his symptoms are not unbearable and the patient can adjust to the constant daytime pit stops and the interrupted sleep at night, then he may very well be advised to wait. As well, a patient's anxiety or concern regarding surgery (which is justifiable, since any operation is potentially dangerous) may be a good reason to continue observation and see if surgery can be avoided.

Dr. Reginald Bruskewitz, Professor of Surgery at the University of Wisconsin, conducted research on more than 500 men with moderate benign prostate enlargement symptoms. The men were randomly assigned to one of two groups. One group underwent surgery (transurethral resection of the prostate, or TURP—see Chapter 6 for more information); the second (control) group did not. Both groups were observed for three to five years. Bruskewitz reported that the men who had surgery had few complications, and all but seven of the nearly 300 men in that group saw improvements in their symptoms after surgery. But the most unexpected finding was that the men who did not have surgery also did very well during the observation period. Dr. Bruskewitz concluded that men with mild symptoms of prostate enlargement probably don't need either surgery or immediate treatment with medication.

Watching for Symptoms

The patient who selects the watchful waiting option should continue regular visits to the doctor and be under observation—

if the problem should persist or get worse, the frequent checkups may save his life. The doctor will probably suggest lifestyle changes during the period of watchful waiting. The patient will be told to urinate regularly (or at least to try!). He will also be advised to avoid drugs or cold medicine that can worsen his condition. Reviewing the regimen for prostatitis in Chapter 2 would be helpful at this point.

The patient should closely observe the behavior of his prostate and alert the doctor if the condition worsens or if new symptoms develop. He should be on the alert for certain symptoms during the period of watchful waiting, as there is the possibility that the enlarged prostate could cause damage to the bladder or kidney. Also, malignant cells may develop during the waiting period and start to spread outside the gland to various parts of the body. If he detects even a hint of urinary retention, the patient should contact his doctor immediately. In the event of recurrent bladder infections, urinary retention, or other symptoms becoming intolerable, the patient may be a logical candidate for more aggressive treatment.

The patient should watch for the following symptoms:

- Slow urine stream and dribbling
- Frequent urination during day and night
- Difficulty in starting or stopping urination
- Painful and burning urination
- Painful ejaculation
- Blood observed in urine or semen
- An aching pain in the penis, scrotum, testicles, anus, lower abdomen, or lower back
- Swollen lymph nodes

If advanced cancer develops, additional symptoms could include fatigue, loss of energy, persistent swelling of one or both lower limbs and back, rib or hip pain, and frequent pain or stiffness in these areas. Sometimes a tumor in the spine can enlarge and squeeze the spinal cord, causing weakness or a numbing feeling in the legs. This is a very serious condition.

Acute Urinary Retention One symptom that requires immediate medical assistance is acute urinary retention. This condition could create a lot of damage to the bladder and kidneys. Under extreme circumstances, it can lead to death.

If complete urinary blockage develops and you cannot void any urine at all, you must see your doctor immediately. The doctor will insert a catheter (a hollow, flexible tube) through the urethra into the bladder in order to drain the urine; this is often referred to as a "ream job." It's a common procedure, but a most unpleasant one. It may only take a minute or two, but it will seem like a lifetime. Medical historians reveal that thousands of years ago, the Egyptians treated this problem by inserting reeds or copper or silver tubes through the penis and urethra to widen the urinary passageway and allow the urine to escape. This primitive and crude catheter probably saved many lives, but it most likely also caused the demise of numerous Egyptians.

If you go through this traumatic experience (as I did), you may start to think more seriously about terminating the watchful waiting period and having a surgical procedure. Yet the prospect of surgery might make you stop and reconsider—just maybe you could wait a little longer.

TESTING DURING WATCHFUL WAITING

One objective during the watchful waiting period is early detection of prostate cancer, should it develop. Early detection can lead to early treatment, making the likelihood of complete recovery relatively high. To this end, your doctor will probably order a PSA test and do a DRE exam on a regular schedule.

If you suddenly have a much higher PSA level, do not panic. When taking the PSA test, as many as one-third of all males over the age of fifty will score higher than 4.0 ng/ml, which is considered by many urologists to be within the suspect zone indicating cancer cells may be present.

But within this group, only about one-third will have detectable prostate cancer. According to one recent survey, when 148 males with elevated PSA levels were examined, researchers found not cancer but enlarged and inflamed prostate tissue as well as a fair number of harmless lumps. Others had high PSA levels because of bicycling (probably due to the pressure the seat puts on the prostate gland). Recent ejaculation was also considered a reason for some high PSA levels. A larger prostate and older age, as we have discussed, will also affect the level.

If the PSA test result shows a much higher level and differs radically from that found in prior years, you may want to ask your doctor if the blood sample was tested by the Ciba Corning method or by the Hybritech's Tandem PSA. The Hybritech's Tandem PSA is currently the only test that is formally approved. If your doctor uses a different type of screening, it can suddenly change the level, causing needless alarm.

It is also possible for a patient to receive someone else's test result. This may sound farfetched, but it happened to me. I received a panic call from my urologist to inform me that my PSA level had soared from the 4 ng/ml level to over 20 ng/ml. Since this figure indicates that malignant cells are present, needless to say, I was very frightened. Subsequent tests taken at a different laboratory were in the 7 ng/ml to 8.8 ng/ml range—not as low as I would have preferred but consistent with the level to be expected in a middle-aged male with an enlarged prostate.

To avoid this problem, you should select a reliable laboratory. One associated with an academic medical center will probably be a good choice. You certainly should have additional tests taken if your PSA level suddenly spurts up to a higher level.

WHEN WATCHFUL WAITING IS NOT APPROPRIATE

You may not have the luxury of opting for deferred maintenance if there is a danger of a large volume of residual urine, decreasing kidney function, bladder stones, other developing bladder problems, or acute urinary retention (a most dangerous condition in which there is complete urinary blockage).

Many types of employment require prolonged urinary retention; therefore watchful waiting is inappropriate. If your job places you in isolated areas far from medical facilities, you may be putting yourself in danger. For example, a forest ranger, lumberjack, or someone who works far from town is at a higher risk of acute complications from prostate problems. This would also apply to fishing and hunting enthusiasts who often hike into the wilderness—unless they take their doctor along on these outings!

Distancing yourself from medical facilities could be disastrous. Consider Howard Hughes, who isolated himself in a room with only his bodyguards; he developed complete urinary retention, which led to kidney failure. If Mr. Hughes had been transported to an emergency hospital or doctor's office immediately, his condition probably could have been treated. It is inexcusable to have something like this happen today.

A PERSONAL ACCOUNT

In my own experience, the decision to wait or to take immediate action was not an easy one to make as the symptoms of my BPH worsened. The quality of my life had definitely been impacted, yet I was very apprehensive about going in for surgery.

The first urologist I visited appeared to be very impatient with me when I asked questions pertaining to my BPH. He suggested that I consider surgery; due to the size of my gland and the symptoms I was experiencing, he believed an operation was inevitable. He was later proved to be correct, but he did not mention any other options, and I perceived that he was too aggressive in wanting to schedule a date for this procedure.

Due to my public health background (as a health educator for the Los Angeles Health Department, a teacher of gerontology, and an author of two books on health), I was well aware of the complications that could develop during surgery. A review of literature pertaining to BPH revealed that the mortality rate of BPH and prostate surgery was less than 1 percent, but I didn't want to be that one out of one hundred. Actually, the cause of death from this operation is usually due to a heart attack or pulmonary problem, and it generally targets patients older than I was.

I decided to get a second opinion. I asked several of my physician friends to whom they would go if they or members of their family had prostate disorders. The name of one particular urologist was mentioned, so I made an appointment with him.

This urologist took the time to explain to me in detail, using diagrams, the progression of my problem and the options for treating it. He outlined a plan of watchful waiting and advised me to call him immediately if I noticed any change in the symptoms, which is what I did.

The most serious problem developed when I experienced urinary retention. The pain, to put it mildly, was excruciating. On the way to the emergency room for some immediate and possibly life-saving treatment, I made up my mind: This is it—no more waiting. If I had any doubts about changing my course of action, the events in the hospital confirmed my decision—never again do I want to go through that much pain. With a great deal of enthusiasm, I looked forward to an operation as soon as possible. But I had to wait about a week for the healing process to take place, during which time a catheter was attached to my leg for the withdrawal of urine. The catheter was finally removed, and an examination showed that I was ready for the operation.

My urologist explained to me, using an enlarged picture of the gland, that my prostate was of a size that required open surgery—an incision through the abdomen. During surgery, the prostatic tissue causing the blockage was removed, and it was found to be nonmalignant. My rehabilitation ran its course, and now I feel as if I have been reborn.

Looking back, I don't regret the problems and inconveniences I subjected myself to during all those years of waiting. I still think it made good sense not to go for surgery until it was definitely necessary, as it turned out to be in my situation. Your situation—or your brother's or your friend's—may be different.

CHAPTER SIX

Considering Surgery

During the period of watchful waiting, a man's condition may improve or he may adjust to getting up two to three times a night. An attitude of submission might now be present: "If this is the worst thing that happens to me, I can handle it." On the other hand, the man's prostate gland may continue to enlarge until the quality of his life becomes intolerable. At this point, surgery may become a more appealing option and may be considered very seriously.

This chapter will cover the issues that a man needs to consider before deciding to have surgery. If the patient has made the decision to be treated surgically, then he will need to choose a urologist to perform the operation, and he should know the different types of procedures that are available. This chapter will cover those crucial topics as well.

SURGERY PROS AND CONS

How can a man evaluate the benefits and risks of surgery? Many in the medical field are still not certain as to what the advantages of an operation on the prostate are. There is a lot of information, including medical studies, available to guide the patient. But every patient is unique, and doctors can offer no universal advice as to which direction to follow. An overwhelming number of urologists have expressed concern for their patients, who must endure much grief from a gland that causes more distress than just about any other structure in the body. Out of this concern, they may recommend surgery, as many urologists share the opinion that an operation on the prostate is one of the few types of surgery that can bring about dramatic improvement in the quality of a patient's life.

Dr. John Weinberg, a researcher at Dartmouth Medical School, looked at the practice styles of urologists in Maine who treated BPH patients. He found that many of the doctors recommended surgery in the belief that it would prevent more serious problems and increase the patient's longevity and quality of life. In fact, the men who had surgery had a slightly decreased life expectancy. The real value of prostate surgery related to the improvement in the quality of the patient's life.

Most patients expect too much from an operation on their prostate gland. Doctors should inform the patient that the objective of the surgery is to reestablish correct functional emptying of the bladder. Even under the best circumstances—the utmost in patient cooperation and the finest surgery and care—the patient may continue to have moderate symptoms for a while. Nocturia, for example, is not going to disappear right away—it will take time to break the habit of frequent nightly trips to the bathroom.

Potential dangers do accompany surgery. I'll review these slight (but real) dangers in detail below. Most urologists agree that the dangers associated with surgery for BPH are grossly exaggerated.

A more legitimate fear concerns the possibility of developing retrograde ejaculation after surgery for BPH. In a healthy male with an erect penis, the bladder neck tightens and forces semen to flow through the penis at ejaculation. Prostate surgery often upsets the bladder neck mechanism and causes retrograde ejaculation, in which the semen flows backward into the bladder and not forward through the penis (semen tends to take the path of least resistance). The sensation is the same, and the semen is released with the next passage of urine. Some men find dry orgasms disturbing. However, no medical danger is associated with retrograde ejaculation. There is a problem only if a man wants to father a child, in which case he can consult his doctor for a technique to resolve this difficulty.

If you do decide to have surgery, then you must select a urologist in whom you have complete confidence. After all, this procedure will have a major impact on your health and wellbeing. We are talking about the rest of your life.

SELECTING A UROLOGIST

You should select a urologist who is not only highly competent but also gentle and compassionate—these are not traits that you will find in all surgeons, but such able and supportive professionals are out there.

James Lewis, an author and a survivor of prostate cancer, suggests calling the urology department at a large hospital and asking the secretary whom he or she would want within the department to operate on a relative (secretaries often learn which doctor is considered the best or most trusted in the hospital).

Ask your primary care physician and friends for their recommendations, especially if they are in the medical profession. Surgical nurses are also a good source of advice.

The local medical society can assist you in obtaining names of urologists you can contact and interview. You can also locate urologists by calling the State Medical Directory, the American Board of Certified Specialists, or the American Medical Association Directory.

In interviewing urologists, find out what type of surgery they generally recommend to relieve your problem (the next section will cover the different types of surgery). Ask about the urologist's proficiency with the nerve-sparing technique (see Chapter 9), which reduces the possibility of becoming impotent. You should also ask how many such operations the urologist has performed and how many patients have experienced adverse side effects.

An operation for BPH isn't as radical as an operation for prostate cancer, but if your doctor discovers malignant tissue during the surgery or after the tissue is removed and analyzed, then you will require additional surgery or treatment. You want to be sure that your urologist is trained to do whatever is necessary.

TYPES OF SURGERY FOR BPH

There are several types of surgery to consider. Your surgeon may lean toward one approach due to his experience and training. Feel free to ask about the reasons for such a surgical preference. After all, it is your body and your dime, and knowledge is power. By discussing openly all aspects of the surgery, you will feel less apprehensive about your hospitalization, which could contribute to a speedier recovery.

There are special circumstances that will rule out one type of surgery and require another. For example, if the estimated size of the prostate tissue is much over 50 grams (about 10 percent of BPH patients fall into this category), then there is difficulty in scraping out that much tissue and drawing it out of the urethra, so an "open" surgical approach (one requiring an incision) is used. One of the open surgical approaches may be used even for a small prostate. If there is a need for the surgeon to remove bladder stones and bladder hernias (diverticula), they can be repaired at the same time.

Transurethral Resection of the Prostate (TURP)

The most common type of prostate surgery, which is used by 90 percent of urologists, is a transurethral resection of the prostate, or TURP. In America, 400,000 men a year get a TURP. It is, next to cataract surgery, the most common operation performed on men who are sixty years of age or older.

The TURP is called a closed operation, as no incision is made. The TURP, regarded as the standard by many doctors, is often called "roto-rapturing" the gland. This type of reference doesn't present an encouraging mental picture for the patient—who wants to compare his operation to that of a snake-like pipe inserted in the toilet bowl to clear obstructions?

American men may feel encouraged to hear of experiments in England in which robots actually perform TURPs. I doubt that many men would stand in line waiting for their turn, but it has actually been performed. Further investigation is underway to see if robot-performed procedures could be the way to handle the backlog of males with BPH problems.

In the standard TURP, which takes about an hour, the doctor inserts a thin hose-like device, called a resectoscope, into the penis.

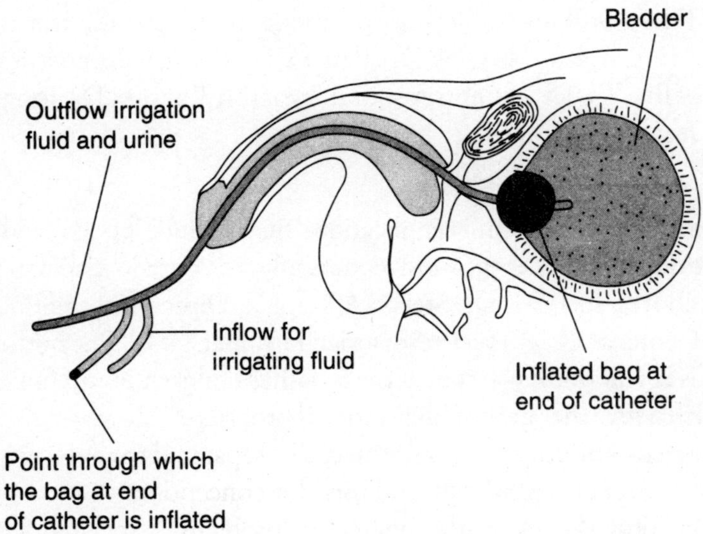

FOLEY CATHETER

Immediately following the TURP procedure, a Foley catheter is placed through the urethra into the bladder.

The patient does not feel any pain, as he is usually under either a local or a spinal-block anesthesia. If you have had arthroscopic work performed by an orthopedic surgeon, you will be familiar with this instrument. The resectoscope has a fiber-optic light source that guides an electrically heated needle to the prostate tissue that is causing the problems. The surgeon then scoops the tissue out, leaving only a shell of the prostate.

A representative sample of the tissue is given to a pathologist, who analyzes it to see if any cancer is present and, if so, what kind. If no cancer is present—good news—the blockage should no longer be a problem. (The bad news is that an absence of cancer at the time doesn't necessarily mean that cancer won't develop eventually—but there are no guarantees in life.) After even a successful TURP, the urologist will probably advise the patient to continue with annual checkups and possibly have more frequent exams. But at least now he can get a good night's sleep and get his exercise in ways other than walking back and forth to the bathroom.

"There is remarkable improvement in symptoms, and the operation is safe," asserts Dr. Patrick C. Walsh. "Almost four out of five TURP patients respond favorably," agrees Dr. Joseph E. Oesterling.

Concerns Long-term complications may include poor bladder control, impotence, or, most commonly, retrograde ejaculation (see above). In 1993, Dr. Steven A. Kaplan, Director of the Prostate Center at Columbia Presbyterian Hospital, said, "The bottom line is if you think you may want to father children in the future, an alternative therapy might be more appropriate." However, there is now a procedure whereby sperm can be separated from the urine after retrograde ejaculation and used for conception.

Dr. John Weinberg also points out problems associated with the TURP. Beginning in 1988, in separate studies of TURP patients, he discovered the following:

- Twenty percent of patients who had moderate symptoms before surgery were unimproved after surgery.
- Twenty percent of patients needed a second TURP operation within ten years of the first operation. The likelihood of tissue regrowth is especially high among the younger age group because they will most likely live many years after the operation. For senior citizens, it is doubtful that they will ever need a second operation.
- Twenty-five percent of patients had short-term complications of varying severity following surgery.
- Four percent ended up with persistent incontinence after surgery.
- Five percent were impotent.
- Up to 25 percent said they were dissatisfied with the results.

But perhaps Dr. Weinberg's most troubling finding related to premature death. He found that TURP patients were more likely to die from heart attacks within five years of surgery than patients who underwent open prostatectomies (see below), a riskier procedure than TURPs. Urologists are at a loss to explain this finding.

Dr. Weinberg's research raised doubts about surgery for some physicians. They recognized the great gaps in their knowledge and became less confident in the outcome of this procedure. It raised all kinds of red flags. The surgical recurrence rate was a shocking revelation. Spurred by these findings, the American Urological Association and federal health officials at the Agency for Health Care Policy and Research formed a panel to review the scientific literature and establish uniform surgical guidelines.

An analysis of deaths in various age groups was provided in a 1992 article in *American Druggist*: deaths occurred during or following surgery and were due to heart attack, stroke, pneumonia, blood clots, or other causes. In the first six weeks after surgery, out of 1,000 men, four men aged fifty-six to sixty-nine died; seven men aged seventy to seventy-four died; ten men aged seventy-five to seventy-nine died; twenty men aged eighty to eighty-four died; and thirty-four men over age eighty-five died.

Even when the TURP is successful, it involves a hospital stay of five to seven days and a convalescence of at least several weeks. It is expensive not only to the patient but also to the U.S. public health system—the total cost of TURPs is soon expected to top five billion dollars annually.

A study of medical patients who had a TURP performed in the period from 1984 to 1990 found that the number of TURPs performed has been declining since 1987, conceivably due to increasing availability of alternative treatments or to changes in the treatment preferences of patients and their doctors.

Transurethral Incision of the Prostate (TUIP)

The transurethral incision of the prostate, or TUIP, is similar to a TURP. The TUIP is considered an open operation, because incisions are involved. In this relatively simple procedure, a pair of incisions are made on the sides of the bladder neck that closes the bladder off from the urethra. The surgeon does not remove any of the prostate tissue that causes the blockage. If the incision is deep enough, the prostate will spring open, and many cases will not subsequently require prostatic resection.

Often, the typical problems of BPH, such as getting up at night and a reduced urine flow, are improved by a TUIP. The procedure is quicker than a TURP, it causes less blood loss and less risk of retrograde ejaculation (about 15 percent), and it has a 1 percent risk of either incontinence or impotence. This procedure is available for widespread clinical use and is, according to Dr. Joseph E. Oesterling, "The most grossly underused treatment for BPH."

Concerns In some patients, symptoms recur within a few months. In others, relief lasts for several years. The TUIP is not recommended for very enlarged prostates. Of the men undergoing a TUIP, 5 to 10 percent will require a second operation.

Retropubic Prostatectomy

In a retropubic (meaning behind the public bone) prostatectomy, the patient is operated on while lying on his back, and a five-inch incision is made in the lower abdomen. The muscle is separated, and the sac containing the intestines is moved away from the bladder. The surgeon then makes an incision into the prostate gland and removes the tissue causing the urethral obstruction. The tissue is sent to the laboratory to see if any cancer is present. The surgeon closes the prostate capsule with sutures, and the muscle fascia and skin are put back in place and closed with stitches.

The advantage of this type of surgery, which became popular in the 1940s, is that it provides a better view of the prostate gland and the bladder neck. This helps to control bleeding after the problem tissue is taken out. Since the bladder itself is not opened, there is no need for a catheter coming through the bladder wall following surgery, as in the suprapubic approach (see below).

The lesser violation of the body offers less potential for problems and is conducive to speedier recovery. Since this technique causes less stress to the patient, it is the preferred choice by most urologists. It is also used when the prostate tissue is too large to be removed by a TURP.

Concerns Obese men and those with a particularly narrow or bony pelvis are not likely candidates for this approach, as it is difficult for the surgeon to have good exposure of the prostate gland.

Suprapubic Prostatectomy

In a suprapubic (above the pubic bone) prostatectomy, an incision about five inches long is made through the abdomen and into the bladder. After the bladder is exposed, the surgeon reaches inside the bladder, pushing an index finger through the bladder neck and down into the prostatic urethra. Then the process of removing the BPH tissue begins. There are two ways to remove the tissue: the blind approach and the visual approach.

Blind Approach The blind approach is so named because the surgeon does the operation by feel alone. With this surgical approach the doctor's finger is inserted into the bladder after it is opened, then into the prostatic urethra, at which point he can start to remove the BPH tissue.

At the end of the operation, a Foley catheter (a latex or silicone tube that drains the urine from the bladder to an outside collection bag) is inserted into the penis opening. The catheter has a water-filled balloon on the bladder end to keep it in place. It continuously drains the urine into a sterile collection bag. It is usually left in for about a week. It may make the patient feel that he has to urinate or it may cause painful bladder spasms (how well I remember asking my wife and other visitors to leave the room until the spasm pain went away). The pain lasts for only a little while—it helps to remember that before long all this pain will be history and the nightmare will end.

An additional catheter is inserted to provide better urine drainage for the first few days after surgery. With two catheters to drain the blood and the urine, the likelihood of clot formation plugging both catheters is minimized. The doctor will remove the bladder tube that is coming through the abdominal wall when the drainage from both catheters is almost free of blood.

With the urethral catheter still in place, the opening into the bladder where the catheter had been closes in about a day or two, after which the urethral catheter can be removed. In about ten days, the urine will become clear of blood and the patient can finally go home.

Concerns The major disadvantage of the blind approach is that there are difficulties controlling bleeding, since the bleeding vessels cannot be seen. This approach also cannot be used for a patient with prostate cancer.

Visual Approach When the visual (or open) approach is used, the incision is made considerably closer to the bladder neck so that the surgeon can see the bladder neck and thus control bleeding after the problematic prostate tissue is removed. Many physicians prefer this approach over the blind approach—they can do a neater repair of the denuded bladder neck in the area where the tissue was removed. In other respects, the visual approach is very similar to the blind approach. The procedures following surgery are basically the same.

Perineal Prostatectomy

This procedure is another kind of open surgery, and has been around the longest of the five types. It involves an incision between the anus and scrotum, allowing the doctor access to the prostate gland from below. It is seldom used today, for there is great danger that the nerve bundles that control the ability to achieve erection will be damaged. It is rare that a man will choose this operation with this high risk when there are so many other ways to resolve the problem. If you think that surgery for enlarged prostates is something new, this type of operation has the distinction of being the oldest type of operation recorded in medical journals. It was used to remove bladder stones before the time of Christ. One can't help but speculate what percentage of patients were cured of their complications and how many did not survive the operation. After all, they did not have access to the medical technology that we enjoy today.

IN A WORD: RESEARCH

So you have several choices. Visit a medical center resource library, if one is available, or the public library, and read as much information as you can to help you understand the various options for treatment. Your urologist can determine which type is most appropriate to relieve the symptoms of your enlarged prostate (and that's just one more reason why it is so important to make the right choice in selecting your urologist). Unfortunately, most of us spend less time choosing a doctor than we do purchasing a car.

CHAPTER SEVEN

Nonsurgical Treatments

Many men with Benign Prostatic Hyperplasia who might benefit from treatment just do not relish the thought of having surgery. Also, many men are not prime candidates for an operation due to their age or medical condition. Fortunately, there are alternative forms of treatment.

Let us look at the variety of options that are available to the male suffering from an enlarged prostate.

BALLOON DILATION

Balloon dilation is one of the newer treatments used at larger medical centers. This technique was first developed by radiologists and cardiologists to perform a coronary angioplasty: a small balloon is inflated inside a blocked coronary artery, "squishing" the blockage and thus widening the vessel, allowing more blood to bring vital oxygen to the heart. The balloons used for enlarging a constricted urethral passage are larger than the ones used by cardiologists.

The technique involves passing a catheter through the urethra, which is being squeezed by the enlarged prostate gland that surrounds it. When the device is positioned at the site of obstruction, the balloon is inflated to push back the prostate tissue and allow the urine to flow more easily through the urethra.

Positioning of the catheter must be precise, for when the balloon is inflated it exerts enormous pressure. If it is inflated inside the bladder, it is simply ineffective. But if it is inflated below the urinary sphincter, incontinence or impotence can result.

This procedure can be done under fluoroscopic control, which is a form of radiation physics, with the patient sedated and with local anesthesia in the urethra. Urologists who use the technique favor it because the local anesthetic makes it easier to perform and places less stress on the patient. It is cost-effective and carries a lower risk of retrograde ejaculation than the TURP procedure (see Chapter 6). Patients are often able to return to their normal occupation the day after the procedure, which is a big plus. For many patients, however, a catheter has to remain in place for another two days.

At an American Urological Association meeting in 1991, a discussion of various studies on balloon dilation was presented, illustrating the many and varied opinions of urologists who use this technique. It appears that the safety of the procedure has been confirmed but its efficiency has not. According to *Hospital Practice* magazine, the reputation of balloon dilation among urologists has fallen considerably from its early heights, and its use appears to have diminished considerably.

German doctors using the process were of the opinion that balloon dilation seemed to lose its effectiveness over time. Fifty-four percent of patients were satisfied with results after six months. Only 34 percent were satisfied after a year. Only 31 percent saw urine flow increase into the normal range, and pressure in the bladder—that urgency to urinate—was rarely reduced.

In another investigation, seventy-four balloon dilation patients were followed for a year or more and had an overall increase in urine flow of only 40 percent. It appeared that younger patients had the best results. A similar result was noted by University of

Iowa physicians who followed thirty-four patients for a year and reported that urination improved right after dilation but the benefits tapered off by the end of a year.

Balloon dilation is not for everyone, and patient selection is important. Men with very large prostates (weighing over 30 to 40 grams) are not good candidates; it is generally agreed that only men with a relatively small prostate gland are good candidates. This technique appeals to patients who do not want to opt for surgery, and the procedure can be very useful for older men and for those with medical conditions that make them poor candidates for conventional surgery.

Many urologists do not recommend this procedure, as it may need to be repeated—about 50 percent of balloon dilation patients experience a return of symptoms within a year. If they do not experience problems within this period, however, there is a good chance that this treatment will have worked for them. The long-term success of this procedure does not appear to approach that of surgery. There is also a 4 percent risk of impotence, a 3 percent risk of incontinence, and a 5 percent risk of retrograde ejaculation.

MICROWAVE THERAPY

In microwave therapy, energy is delivered by an antenna inside a catheter, which can heat prostate tissue over a period of time, allowing a more normal flow of urine. It is still debatable as an effective treatment for BPH.

There are several types of equipment in use or being developed to deliver heat to the prostate gland in order to slowly shrink the enlarged gland without damaging the surrounding tissue.

Prostatron

A heat-generating microwave machine called the Prostatron has been used extensively in France (where it was developed) and in England. Since 1991, it has been used to treat over 30,000 patients. The machine costs around a quarter of a million dollars and consequently is not something you can expect to find in a urologist's office.

With the Prostatron method, first the size of the patient's prostate gland is evaluated. Then a treatment catheter with a tiny internal antenna is inserted into the urethra and positioned at the center of the prostate with a small ultrasound probe. The Prostatron heats the prostate gland while a cooling system keeps the urethra from being damaged. The unwanted tissue is destroyed by the microwave heat and slowly absorbed by the body over the course of a few weeks.

By this time, the tissue should shrink so that the urine can flow freely. Retrograde ejaculation, a problem associated with surgery and other forms of treatment, is not likely to result.

Physicians at the Prostate Unit in the Department of Urology of Charing Cross Hospital in London, England, recently reported their results using the Prostatron. The average patient was sixty-seven years old and had significant symptoms of prostate enlargement, such as urine retention and obstruction of the urethra. Some of the men were given a fake treatment, while the others received microwave therapy.

Those treated with the Prostatron had a 70 percent decrease in symptoms, a 53 percent increase in urinary flow rate, and a 92 percent decrease in the residual urine in the bladder after urination. For the men in the control group, there was no real improvement.

One complication noted was a 22 percent increase in acute retention of urine in the microwaved group that was limited to the immediate posttreatment period. One patient continued to have posttreatment retention that had not resolved in ten days, and he decided to go for surgery.

A six-month study of 150 men aged forty-three to eighty-three with enlarged prostates at five medical centers in 1991 produced overall favorable results with the Prostatron. Although 36 percent of the patients required urinary catheterization, all were free of the catheters by the six-week follow-up. Researchers concluded that the study demonstrates the safety, effectiveness, patient tolerability, and durability of transurethral microwave thermotherapy. Retrograde ejaculation or sexual dysfunction were rare side effects of the therapy. (In comparison, surgery relieves symptoms somewhat more effectively, but it also causes medically significant side effects.)

Dr. Joseph E. Oesterling of the University of Michigan compared the effectiveness of three methods of increasing urine flow and found the following: drugs increase the urine flow by up to 2 millimeters per second; the Prostatron increases it by 4 millimeters per second, and surgery increases urine flow by 6 millimeters per second. Based on this, Oesterling believes the device may indeed fill that gray zone between drugs and surgery.

Transrectal Microwave Thermal Therapy

This method involves inserting a microwave probe into the rectum to destroy the prostate tissue that is obstructing the flow of urine. The destroyed tissue is then carried off via the urine. A definite advantage of this over the TURP is that it can be performed on an outpatient basis. It requires only a local anesthetic.

One disadvantage is that in order to destroy the targeted prostate tissue without impairing the adjacent structure, it is necessary for the patient to have three to ten low-dosage treatments. This does not appeal to most patients, who generally prefer a one-time procedure. Urologists generally recommend transurethral microwave thermal therapy as a more effective and convenient treatment.

ULTRASOUND

In the ultrasound procedure, ultrasound waves are used to turn the prostate tissue into pulp, which is then sucked out of the body by aspiration. A general or spinal anesthetic is required, and the procedure performed in the hospital.

This technique causes less blood loss than does surgical removal of the enlarged portions of the prostate gland, and it involves a much lower incidence of retrograde ejaculation. The jury is still out as to its overall desirability.

LASER SURGERY

This treatment involves inserting a laser probe into the prostatic urethra to vaporize tissue. It is done quickly, avoiding the trauma often associated with surgery. Compared with a TURP, laser surgery causes almost no bleeding, requires less anesthesia, and results in less incontinence.

The disadvantage is that relief is not immediate. Destroyed tissue must be sloughed off through the urine, which takes two to six weeks. The laser does not remove tissue instantly, so a catheter is used for a short period of time after the treatment. Many urologists want to see the long-term results before they use laser surgery instead of the TURP.

As with other methods of treatment, laser surgery is not for everyone. Patients with an extremely large prostate or with prostate cancer are not candidates for this technique. Patient selection begins with a careful examination by the urologist.

Most surgeons agree that lasers, which are already in use, will play a growing role in treating BPH in the future. But they say that more information is needed before they can determine who is a suitable candidate for the procedure, what the optimal energy level and duration of laser use are, and whether ultrasound guidance is really needed.

A study of 235 patients at ten medical centers, using the laser procedure, was initiated in 1990, and it was reported on at the meeting of the American Urological Association. Men in the study showed an average of 69 percent improvement in their urine flow, and a 67 percent improvement in overall symptoms. Their average hospitalization was 1.4 days, with 85 percent of the patients either staying overnight or going home the same day.

Compared with traditional surgery, laser surgery is cost-effective and requires less anesthesia, medication, and time. Other advantages include minimal blood loss, shorter convalescence, and no reported serious complications. A 1992 announcement from the Stanford University Medical Center stated that patients who underwent laser surgery for BPH could go home immediately after the half-hour procedure.

Several years later, the same enthusiasm for this process is expressed further by researchers at Stanford University, who claim that one treatment of BPH by this process is just as effective and safer than the popular TURP.

The outcome of using a Neodymium Yag laser to burn away the excess tissue was most impressive. Of the 227 men who received this treatment in one study, 85 to 90 percent showed considerable improvement in ease of urination. This is comparable to results obtained with the TURP, which is considered the gold standard by many surgeons.

Transurethral Ultrasound Laser Incision of the Prostate (TULIP)

This technology is for treating noncancerous enlargement of the prostate. It has been developed by Dr. Robert Roth, a Lahey Clinic urologist, in conjunction with Intra-Sonix, Inc. of Burlington, Massachusetts. It uses a miniature ultrasound device to guide the laser to the site of prostate obstruction inside the urethra, where it can heat and distroy excess prostate tissue. It causes no bleeding, which eliminates the need for irrigating fluid that can cause heart and lung complications following traditional surgery.

Visual Laser Ablation of the Prostate (VLAP)

This technique involves inserting a microscope and a laser into the urethra. The laser heats the prostate tissue, which is slowly eliminated, relieving the symptoms of BPH.

The advantages are that it can be done on an outpatient basis with local anesthesia. There is very little risk of impotence, incontinence, or retrograde ejaculation.

STENTS

A stent is a spring-like device composed of self-anchoring metal mesh tubes that is placed into the prostatic urethra, where it is left on a temporary or semipermanent basis. It is used to stretch the channel within the prostatic urethra so that the patient can have an easier time in urinating. For a small number of patients with chronic urinary retention problems who are not candidates for surgery due to heart or lung disease or other conditions, stents may be a helpful option. They are often recommended as a short-term solution for elderly men who are poor candidates for surgery due to ill health. Stents are used by urologists in England and Scandinavia. They can be inserted quickly and easily on an outpatient or overnight basis, with no blood loss.

The outcome of this procedure has been fair, with slightly more than half having satisfactory results. Unfortunately, prostate tissue may grow through the mesh and block the urethra again, making a surgical procedure necessary. Instead of the spring-like device, some urologists have tried using stainless steel stents, but the results have been similar.

MEDICATION

Some physicians will treat their patients with one of several drugs that relax the smooth muscle surrounding the prostate. The entire prostate gland may then relax and expand outward slightly, presumably allowing the channel of the prostatic urethra to open. This decreases the volume of tissue that is obstructing the flow of urine and causing so much discomfort, and the urine is able to flow.

Dibenzyline

Drugs widely used to control high blood pressure and to remove urethral obstructions that reduce normal flows have been found helpful in treating the enlarged prostate. One example is Dibenzyline. This drug has been used for years to lower high blood pressure. As little as 10 milligrams of Dibenzyline a day doubled the urine flow in 46 percent of the patients studied over a ten-year period, and 80 percent were relieved of obstructive symptoms.

Some physicians are skeptical, however, and claim that Dibenzyline causes cancer in the digestive tract of rats. Nasal obstruction, delay or inhibition of orgasm, and a significant danger of lowering the patient's blood pressure are cited as other reasons to avoid its use. Further study is necessary, but if the problems related to its use can be ameliorated, then it could be another valuable tool to help the patient.

Flutamide (Euxelin), Casodex, and Zeness

Flutamide, sold under the name Euxelin, is receiving a lot of interest as a drug to control "bad testosterone." There are two categories of testosterone: "good" testosterone is manufactured in the testicles; "bad" testosterone, or dihydrotestosterone (DHT), is produced inside the prostate from the testosterone furnished by the testicles. DHT is necessary in order for the male to enjoy normal physical development at puberty. But as he grows older, it creates problems by causing excess tissue to grow in the prostate.

Flutamide is intended to inhibit the production of DHT inside the prostate without preventing the good testosterone from doing its job in other parts of the body. It appears to be working for many patients. There are side effects, but not usually severe ones: patients have experienced gastrointestinal problems and, very rarely, some problems associated with the liver.

In October 1995, the pharmaceutical company Zeneca, Inc. received FDA clearance to use Casodex, a new antiandrogen (a medication that reduces or eliminates the presence or activity of androgens) for the hormonal treatment of advancing prostate cancer. Its objective is to reduce the production of the male hormone testosterone and to block stimulation of prostate cancer cells by any remaining testosterone. It was tested as part of a treatment regimen called maximal androgen blockade (MAB) on 813 patients with advanced prostate cancer.

The most commonly reported adverse effects as reported in a study by Dr. Paul Schellhammer and colleagues were hot flashes (49 percent), general pain (27 percent), constipation (17 percent), back pain (15 percent), asthenia (13 percent), pelvic pain (13 percent), nausea (11 percent), diarrhea (10 percent), and infection (10 percent).

Recently, Casodex and a similar drug, Zeness, have come on the market. They are antiandrogens that work similarly to Flutamide by blocking a cell's ability to absorb hormones. A patient only has to take one pill a day, but in some patients it causes gastrointestinal difficulties.

Proscar (Finasteride)

Proscar is receiving a lot of attention as a possible solution to prostate problems. Manufactured by Merck and Co., Inc., it is generically known as Finasteride. The story behind the development of Proscar is fascinating and almost reads like a Hollywood film script. Scientists at Merck had made a commitment to develop a drug to treat the symptoms of BPH as early as 1966. A plan was put into action to study endocrine approaches to BPH. The initial plan was to focus on the development of antiantigen or antiprogesterone agents to help interrupt the growth of the prostate.

By the end of the decade, it was generally believed that DHT, rather than testosterone, was the key hormone involved in the growth of the prostate gland, and 5-alpha reductase, the enzyme that catalyzes the conversion of testosterone to DHT, had been described. At this time, scientists began to consider reorienting their prior research to focus on DHT-antagonists (DHT-inhibitors) and on 5-alpha reductase.

Then the plot thickened. Scientists observed a group of males on a small Caribbean island who had a congenital deficiency of 5-alpha reductase at birth and were raised as girls. But at puberty they started to develop male genitals, hair on the face and other parts of the body, and an interest in females. The adult males who had genetically inhibited 5-alpha reductase showed decreased levels of DHT, had small prostate glands, and—most significantly—did not develop BPH. They also did not have normal beard growth, acne, or chronological hair growth.

Based on these findings, it was theorized that a specific inhibitor of 5-alpha reductase might have the potential to shrink an enlarged prostate without affecting testosterone-dependent functions or causing other adverse reactions.

You can just imagine the excitement this revelation must have caused for the investigators at Merck research laboratories. Scientists pursued the development of inhibitors to 5-alpha reductase and developed a class that would show the growth of the prostate.

One of these compounds, Finasteride, was found to be effective in treating enlarged prostates in dogs, and it was later used on humans. Trials of Finasteride began in 1986, and it was approved by the FDA in 1992. Will this be the magic bullet that will end so much suffering and pain among so many American males? It could very well be, but as with many drugs, it does have a downside. A major drawback to the use of Proscar is that it takes about three months before the prostate shrinks enough to help in urinary flow problems, and for the prostate sufferer this can seem like a lifetime.

Proscar also reduces a man's level of prostate-specific antigen (PSA); a low value usually indicates that a man is less likely to have cancer than men with higher levels. But when the PSA level has been reduced by Proscar, it complicates the diagnosis. According to Jerome P. Pichie, Professor of Surgery at Harvard and Chief of Urology at Brigham and Women's Hospital, "Men should have a PSA test before starting Proscar and another one three to six months later." If a man's PSA levels have not dropped by one-third to one-half after taking the drug for several months, this may signal the presence of prostate cancer or another problem. In this case, a urologist should be consulted to investigate further.

An article in the April 12, 1995, issue of *The Wall Street Journal* quoted a representative of Merck and Co., Inc., as saying, "Proscar may grow hair on bald men's heads, so if it doesn't prove to be the wonder drug for shrinking the prostate, the investment in the drug may still be profitable." Merck has high hopes for this drug and expects it to generate a billion-dollar profit.

An article in *The American Druggist* lists the pros and cons of taking Proscar. The one advantage listed is:

- Improvement of symptoms: After one year, symptoms improve to some degree in 63 percent of men.

The three disadvantages listed are:

- Slow action: Patients may have to wait six months to a year for the drug to work.
- Impotence: Within one year, 4 percent of men have some trouble having an erection.
- Decreased ejaculate: Within a year, 3 percent of men have a decrease in semen produced.

Although preliminary results look favorable, investigators will have to look at the long-term effect of this medication as it relates to the prostate and its effect on the development of prostate cancer.

Hytrin

Hytrin is another drug considered as an alternative to surgery for the correction of prostate problems. An article in *Drug Topics* states that Hytrin relaxes the smooth muscle around the bladder neck and prostate. This lessens the pressure on the urethra and helps the urine to flow more regularly. The drug takes about two weeks to work, and in clinical trials it has improved urine flow and relieved related symptoms of BPH in about 70 percent of users. So far, the drug has been shown to continue working for as long as 30 months. A small number of patients may not be able to tolerate it or may not show an improvement.

Hytrin does have side effects, including dizziness, drowsiness, blurry vision, nausea, and some swelling of the feet or hands. The drug lowers the blood pressure of patients with high blood pressure, but it has minimal impact on patients with normal blood pressure. Hytrin does not affect PSA values.

Doxazosin (Cardura)

Dr. David F. Marley, attending urological surgeon at Memorial Hospital in Houston, Texas, stated at the 89th annual American Urological Association meeting in 1994 that he had found the drug Doxazosin (Cardura, manufactured by Pfizer) to be safe and effective.

Cardura is designed to relax small muscles in the arteries and thus lower blood pressure, effectively relaxing the prostate. It is now FDA-approved. In about a third of cases studied, Cardura dramatically improved the flow rate of urine and significantly decreased symptoms such as urgency and frequency. One side effect: 15 percent of the men experienced dizziness and vertigo.

The Agency for Health Care Policy and Research (AHCPR) recently published clinical practice guidelines on the diagnosis and treatment of BPH. The AHCPR guidelines listed alpha-blockers, including Doxazosin, as effective treatments for this common condition.

Leuprolide (Lupron)

Leuprolide is a drug that is being used experimentally to shrink the prostate. It reduces the testosterone to about the level that castration does, resulting in the prostrate gland shrinking, but the side effects are significant and impotence was caused in some men who were sexually active prior to taking the injections. The jury is still out as to its value; studies have shown that half of the men treated with it still had symptoms associated with an enlarged prostate. It is not known to cause any toxic effects, but it has not received clinical support. It is also rather expensive.

Bee Pollen and Other "Natural" Drugs

Bee pollen provides a mixture of amino acids, vitamins, minerals, and enzymes. In addition to claims that it improves the skills of athletes, bee pollen is said to help shrink an enlarged prostate. In some, it may cause a serious allergic reaction. Many males are allured by the tempting offers and testimonials published in many ads and newsletters: "Thank you—it works"; "My wife also appreciates how it cured me and turned our sex life around"; "To think of how long I suffered needlessly"; "Greater flow of urine"; "No more pain."

Everyone would love to have access to a magic pill that would eliminate all kinds of pain and suffering, especially when the problem could lead to one's demise. But no such pill exists, and it probably never will. In the meantime, all too many men out of despair are willing to try anything or believe anyone in order to relieve their anxiety and distress.

Clinical verification of the so-called wonder cures has not been provided. In the rare instances where there are apparently verified claims of improvement from macrobiotic diets and other nutritional approaches and nontraditional therapies, it could very well be an example of the placebo effect. In addition to wasting hard-earned money on products that have not been tested and approved by creditable agencies, there are possible dangers associated with using unproven remedies: allergies, urinary irritation, diarrhea, sleeping problems, nervousness, skin irritations, mental disorientation, and, in some cases, even breast enlargement. Several years ago, the U.S. Postal Service challenged many of these products sold through the mail, claiming that they were misleading the public with false advertising, and banned them from the mail. In 1990, the Food and Drug Administration said it would ban the sale of all nonprescription drugs used to treat the prostate gland.

Laetrile Laetrile was touted as a cure for prostate cancer years ago, and it still has many prostate patients heading for Mexico, Spain, and Italy to get this "wonder drug." Clinics sprang up in which doctors (many of them of questionable background) assured patients that they would cure them by giving them this drug.

Laetrile is produced by processing amygdalin, a complex cyanide-containing chemical obtained from the seeds of apricots, peaches, and bitter almonds. The doctors who prescribe this treatment believe that the cyanide in Laetrile distroys malignant cells. The product was never approved for sale in the United States and can only be obtained by smugglers who bring it into the country. The National Cancer Institute has said it is useless and can be dangerous.

It is bad enough that patients may have their hopes built up only to be disappointed, but they can also be exposed to the potential danger of cyanide poisoning, which can cause severe illness or death. Taking Laetrile or eating large quantities of apricots, peach pits, and almonds is not the answer.

Herbs and Natural Remedies Many products are receiving a lot of attention from creditable health investigators. Some medicinal herbs appear to have merit in helping to heal the prostate gland. One in particular that is getting a lot of attention is the saw palmetto berry.

The saw palmetto berry, also called serenoa repens, is native to the United States and was used by the Seminole hundreds of years ago as a potent aphrodisiac. It has gained popularity in Italy over the past quarter century; now, it accounts for 38 percent of all medications prescribed for benign prostatic hyperplasia in that country.

Many European researchers in France and Britain are very optimistic about its use. A study of 110 men with BPH showed that saw palmetto extract significantly increased urine flow, decreased the amount of urine left in the bladder after urinating, and cut down the nighttime excursions to the bathroom. A study in Italy showed similar results.

The herb works by possibly preventing the breakdown of testosterone into phihydrotestosterone (PHT), a more potent form of the hormone that researchers believe may trigger prostate enlargement. Results from a recent clinical study published in the medical journal *Current Therapeutic Research* corroborate numerous other double-blind controlled studies showing that the fat soluble extract of saw palmetto is an effective treatment for BPH. The journal went so far as to say it was superior to any other drug prescribed for BPH.

The FDA outlawed its sale as an over-the-counter prostate treatment in 1990. It can still be sold legally in the U.S. as a food supplement. Since it has no side effects, many are purchasing it. The testing required to have it approved by the FDA as a drug for prostate treatment would cost $200 million, which is too much for a small herb company. The cost is $19.95 for 100 capsules (about a month's supply).

Shark Cartilage

Shark cartilage has been used by an increasing number of patients and clinicians to treat nonresponsive cancer and other degenerative diseases. The FDA has granted an investigational new drug application to Lane Labs USA, Inc., which will conduct a study to determine the effect of using shark cartilage to treat prostate cancer patients and AIDS patients who suffer from Kaposi's sarcoma.

The use of shark cartilage was the focus in 1993 of a *60 Minutes* TV news story; another report later that year focused on a promising human clinical trial conducted in Cuba in which several terminal cancer patients responded positively to shark cartilage therapy. New studies are being conducted to determine its effect on prostate cancer.

Dr. Lane's recommended dosage is half a gram multiplied by the patient's weight. He claims that 7 to 8 grams a day may prevent recurrence of cancer, but he emphasizes that it should be accompanied by proper nutrition and either a traditional or nontraditional treatment for prostate cancer.

Black Tea

Tea, one of the most popular beverages in the world, is often said to provide protection against cancer. However, epidemiological evidence has been inconclusive. A recent investigation of the benefits of black tea does not support the premise that it will protect against four of the major cancers in humans. A cancer-enhancing effect was not evident either.

FINDING A TREATMENT THAT WORKS

There are many who question the activities of the FDA. When evidence shows that a product does not have side effects and offers a safe, effective, and low-cost option for men with BPH, the FDA usually will not approve it. Does pressure come from the established medical community? Or is the FDA swayed by lobbying efforts from the big drug companies? To many it doesn't make sense that some new treatments are developed here and then are shipped to Europe, where men overseas can derive the benefits. A patient should investigate what is out there and discuss it with his doctor, but he should certainly not try to treat himself without the supervision of his physician.

PART III

What to Do If You Have Prostate Cancer

CHAPTER EIGHT

Watchful Waiting

The best type of treatment for a man diagnosed with prostate cancer depends on many factors, including his age, family background, and overall health. The primary factor is the stage the cancer has reached—particularly whether malignant cells have spread outside the prostate gland. At the present time, though, it is impossible to give universal advice and state specifically at what age a person should wait and at what age a person should seek treatment.

CHOOSING THE WATCHFUL WAITING OPTION

Many urologists believe that a man in his late seventies or eighties with a limited life expectancy will most likely die of something else, so there is no need to expose him to treatment that will cause discomfort and pain plus incur considerable financial costs; in this case, the treatments may be more dangerous than the disease. Thus, watchful waiting is a preferred option for this patient.

Mark S. Litwin, Assistant Professor of Urology at UCLA, is studying the quality-of-life issues that face prostate cancer patients; he observes that what is most important to men is not the number of years they have left but the quality of those years. "An eighty-two-year-old man with prostate cancer who is completely potent and sexually active may prefer four years of potent, continent life to six years of impotent, incontinent life," Dr. Litwin observed.

Although many men die without even being aware that they have malignant cells in their prostate, this does not mean that a man with prostate cancer should just go on with his life and neglect the disease. Even if he has a low-grade cancer that is well defined and a low PSA for his age, he should still be monitored on a regular basis.

If, however, the patient has a significant cancer as shown by the results of the PSA test, biopsies, and ultrasound and he has a projected life expectancy longer than ten to twenty years, then the doctor will most likely suggest an operation or treatment appropriate for the stage of the disease.

The decision to wait or to seek treatment is not an easy decision to make, since prostate cancer does not follow the same growth pattern in each person. It behaves differently for each man, and it is almost impossible to compare the treatment between one patient and another.

Information to guide the doctor and patient is certainly needed. Strategies for early detection may cause a great deal of confusion if there are no clear answers about what to do if the patient has prostate cancer.

THE WATCHFUL WAITING DEBATE

To help solve this perplexing dilemma—which is being faced by increasingly more men as the population grows older and better means of detection are developed—a study often referred to as the "Swedish study" began.

In this study, a Swedish team of urologists and cancer epidemiologists came up with valuable data. They studied 223 patients identified as having early stage (grade I) prostatic cancer that was initially untreated. Symptomatic patients with tumor progression were treated with estrogen or by surgical removal of the testicles. If the tumor growth remained localized and metastases were not present, no treatment was given, as was standard practice in Sweden in March 1977 (when the study began). Later, the men who were under seventy-five years of age with moderately or poorly differentiated (grade II or III) tumors were randomly allocated to receive local irradiation or no therapy. Only the latter were included in this study. Patients who were seventy-five years or older were not treated and were also included.

> Only 19 patients (8.5 percent) had died of prostate cancer after a mean follow-up of 123 months (range, 81 to 165), and 105 of a total of 124 deaths were from other causes. The ten-year disease-specific survival was 86.8 percent and 87.8 percent in a subgroup of 58 patients who met current indications for radical prostatectomy. The progression-free ten-year survival was 53.1 percent. In about two-thirds of patients, local growth provided the only evidence of progression, and endocrine therapy was "generally successful" in these cases. (Orth, Gomer K., Unden, A.L., et al. "Social Isolation and Mortality in Ischemic Disease. A Ten-year Follow-up Study of 150 Middle-age Men." *Acta Med. Scand.* (1988: 244[3]), 205–15).

In other words, a lot more men died *with* prostate cancer than *of* it.

Comments by Dr. Ralph deVere White concerning this study are enlightening: "It struck me, having looked through the history of this disease as reported by this study, if 10 percent of patients who had a radical prostatectomy die of the disease and 12 percent of patients who have absolutely no treatment immediately die of the disease, why would anyone ever consider having their prostate cancer treated?"

However, Dr. deVere White believes that the American experience with prostate diseases is different from that reported in the Swedish study. In Sweden, 60 percent of the study group have the very lowest stage of cancer. In looking at the American series of patients who have undergone surgery, the figure is about 10 percent. Since these were vastly different figures, I asked Dr. deVere White what his numbers were. He reviewed the last hundred radical prostatectomies that he performed to see how many of those were like the Scandinavian patients. Only 5 percent of them had that very low malignant type of tumor, compared to the 60 percent reported in the Swedish study.

"Similarly, close to 60 percent of the Swedish study patients are dead of some cause other than prostate cancer in ten years. When you look at surgery series in America, what you see is that at ten and fifteen years in close to 1,000 patients who have been operated on, only 20 percent die of something else. Again, this fact that the patient dies does not mean they did not receive the right treatment, namely none. What it does mean is if you are an average American, you are going to have a more aggressive cancer, you are going to live longer, and therefore you would be foolish to have taken at face value the difference in survival between the American series and the Scandinavian series.

"The final bit of evidence is that we know if patients go and get the cancer in the bones they do not do so well. When one looks at the Scandinavian series, even taking all of the above into account, twice as many of those people develop disease in their bones than in the radical prostatectomy series.... You are not comparing apples and apples, but rather apples and oranges if you just take it on face value."

Sweden also has a socialized medical plan, and the question arises: does the cost of surgery for prostate cancer affect the decision about the type of treatment selected? To watch and wait is considerably less expensive than performing an operation, particularly in the early stages of treatment.

Other Studies

A massive study accumulated data on prostates that were surgically treated between 1981 and 1991; the results were reported on by a group calling itself the Prostate Patient Outcome Research Team. According to lead author Dr. Craig Fleming of Oregon Health Sciences University, the results of the study were evaluated using the figures that came out of the Swedish report as a measuring tool. At least 30 percent of the potent men who underwent prostatectomy in this period became impotent; 7 percent lost all urinary control; and many more had intermittent difficulties in both areas. Twenty percent learned that during surgery the tumor was discovered to have already spread and that they would need further treatment (radiation, hormone therapy, or removal of the testicles).

Two other major studies that added to the controversy over delaying treatment were reported for the Prostate Patient Outcome Research team.

Writing for the team in one report, Dr. Fleming studied the actual outcome of patients who, instead of having a radical prostatectomy, were treated with radiation or watchful waiting. The men who participated in the investigation were fifty to seventy-five years of age and had stage A and B tumors.

Dr. Fleming concluded that watchful waiting is "a reasonable alternative to invasive treatment." He added, "We could find no study or groups of studies in the medical literature that definitively support the benefits of either treatment (radiation or prostatectomy) over watchful waiting.... We are doing a lot in this country, yet it is unclear that we know what we are doing."

It's enough to make a patient on the fence decide to wait it out.

The other study was authored by Dr. Grace Lu-Yao of Dartmouth Medical School, who followed the probable prognoses for men sixty-five years and older who had radical prostatectomies. These were men on Medicare and in various geographic locations. Based on 101,980 radical prostatectomies, Dr. Lu-Yao concluded that little benefits were seen as a result of prostate surgery.

Dr. Lu-Yao's and Dr. Fleming's reports were published in the May 1993 issue of *JAMA* as well as in major newspapers, both suggesting that the benefits of prostate surgery were highly overrated.

To further study the "watch and wait" approach as it applies to male patients with localized cancers, a team of researchers headed by urologist Dr. Gerald W. Chodak, Professor of Surgery at Weiss Memorial Hospital in Chicago, examined 828 case records from six studies published in the last ten years, including Swedish and Israeli investigations. The researchers concluded that for men with a life expectancy of ten years or less, watchful waiting is a reasonable option. But men in their forties or fifties face a different choice: radical surgery may completely cure them, adding twenty or thirty years to their lives; some could live for decades and never need treatment.

"The younger you are, the more there is to gain from treatment. The older you are, the more there is to lose," Dr. Chodak said. "At some point, the lines cross. But that point is different for each patient." Dr. Chodak also commented that the issue is about trade-offs—each option has its own set of risks and benefits; the key is to be informed.

But patients rarely get accurate information about the odds of treatment success and the risk of side effects, Dr. Chodak said. Doctors supply vague or overly optimistic information. Patients don't ask enough questions. "We find more and more people coming to us saying that the minute the doctor told them they had cancer, they've been in a fog ever since," said Robert Kanter, founder of the Cincinnati chapter of Man to Man, a prostate cancer support group.

Dr. Patrick C. Walsh comments that the oft-cited studies were not set up objectively or adequately controlled. The studies did not acknowledge the fact that 60 percent of the patients in the Chodak report had stage D tumors (which had spread outside the gland), whereas at Johns Hopkins only 11 percent of the patients who had a radical prostatectomy had stage D disease.

Dr. Walsh acknowledged that for patients with stage A disease, electing to watch and wait is reasonable. Additional research is needed to help resolve this ongoing controversy.

MAKING AN INFORMED DECISION

Because of the PSA test, the DRE, and the fact that men are living longer, the diagnosis of men with prostate cancer is increasing at a galloping rate. In fact, the number of operations for the disease for Medicare patients jumped sixfold from about 2,600 in 1984, before the use of the PSA test, to about 16,000 in 1990, and the rate keeps growing. Many doctors wonder if this trend is spinning out of control.

Since not all cases of diagnosed cancer are destined to cause symptoms or impact adversely on the life of the patient, selecting which patient requires treatment and what treatment to use remains an area of increasing controversy. Prostate cancer is certainly a challenge for doctors. It is a disease that they have learned to diagnose long before they have a consensus about whether and how to treat it.

In America, we are fortunate that we have the option to decide whether we want to watch and wait, have surgery, or select a different type of treatment.

This is a time for a very serious, in-depth discussion with your doctor to help you make the right choice from the menu of treatment options. As important as such a discussion is, evidently a gap exists between the perceptions of doctors and those of their patients regarding this process. A poll of urologists and men who had been diagnosed with prostate cancer showed that 99 percent of the urologists recalled discussing the options with their patients, but only 85 percent of the patients recalled having their options delineated. Perhaps the patients were so emotionally impacted by the news of having prostate cancer that they could not retain what was said. It's a good idea for a patient to record the doctor's discussion of his condition and then listen to it after he has had some time to adjust to the realization that he has this disease.

CHAPTER NINE

Considering Surgery

When a prostate cancer patient can expect a cure or long-term survival, the preferred treatment of many urologists is total removal of the prostate gland. This is considerably different than the surgery for benign prostatic hyperplasia because, in this case, the entire prostate gland is taken out. The operation for BPH involves removal of only the portion of the prostate gland that is obstructing the flow of urine, leaving behind the true prostate tissue (the substance of the normal prostate gland) and the true capsule of the prostate.

Just as there are different surgical methods for relieving the symptoms associated with an enlarged prostate, there are two methods for operating on a cancerous prostate: radical retropubic surgery and radical perineal surgery. The physician will discuss these methods with the patient.

The urologist will select the method that he or she feels is best for the patient and the one that he or she is most skilled at and can perform with the fewest complications. Either form of surgery will take two to four hours. A third surgical procedure—the orchiectomy—does not directly involve the prostate, but it is a related operation and will be discussed briefly below.

RADICAL RETROPUBIC SURGERY

The most common method used in this country is the retropubic approach; as you recall in Chapter 6, "BPH: Considering Surgery," it is preferred by urologists for relieving BPH problems when the prostate gland is too large for a TURP. Many doctors think that it is the most logical approach, as it permits the removal and examination of the pelvic lymph nodes to which the prostate cancer tends to spread.

For this approach, the doctor makes an incision from just below the belly button to the top of the pubic bone. This part of the procedure is the same as that for BPH. The big difference is that in the BPH operation, only the portion of the gland that was obstructing the flow of urine and causing annoyance is removed; most of the prostate tissue and the capsule are left behind. However, a total prostatectomy removes your cancerous prostate completely—and also the seminal vesicles that lie along the prostate (they are the two glands that provide nutrients to the semen).

A cancer that is confined to the prostate gland can usually be eliminated by this procedure. If the cancer is discovered to have spread to the lymph nodes, then the operation will not continue. Other types of therapy, such as hormone treatment, will probably be more effective in such a case.

There is often a considerable loss of blood from this type of surgery. Recovery requires ten days to two weeks, and involves insertion of a catheter, which will be removed in about three weeks.

RADICAL PERINEAL SURGERY

The other surgical option for removing the prostate gland is called the radical perineal approach. You may recall that this procedure was also used for the relief of BPH. The incision is made through the perineum, which is between the scrotum and anus.

Many doctors prefer this method, as they feel that it is less stressful to the patient and that it is easier to perform unless the patient is obese (which makes it difficult because of the large abdominal wall).

A major drawback is that it is difficult to use the nerve-sparing technique (see below) with the perineal approach. Another disadvantage is that it is not possible to examine or remove any of the lymph nodes to which the prostate cancer may have spread. This makes it impossible to know whether to proceed with a radical prostatectomy.

This approach is favored by some urologists because the postoperative effects are much easier on the patient: an abdominal incision is considerably more uncomfortable than a perineal incision.

ORCHIECTOMY

Orchiectomy is removal of the testicles. This operation may be recommended in stage D prostate cancer, when the cancer has spread too far to be operable. Removal of the testicles is a means to lower the level of testosterone in an effort to slow the spread of the cancer.

The advantage of an orchiectomy is that it is relatively simple and effective, and it is performed only once. It requires only a local anesthetic, and the patient can usually go home the day of the surgery. There is usually only minor pain or soreness for a few days.

The dangers of orchiectomy include a risk of infection and the possibility of bleeding following the surgery. And although the orchiectomy will lessen the symptoms, it is not curative; the cancer remains. However, the pain from the cancer will often disappear, and sometimes the patient will notice a dramatic diminishing of pain within a few days.

SELECTING A SURGEON

You should choose your surgeon carefully. The advice provided in Chapter 6 about how to select a urologist is applicable here.

In addition, question any potential urologist about their specific experience in performing operations for the removal of prostate cancer.

Avoid doctors who do not know the nerve-sparing technique (see below), who have performed fewer than 150 prostatectomies, or who have patients with higher rates of incontinence and impotence than those reported in journal articles by surgeons from major teaching hospitals. According to a Johns Hopkins newsletter, a rate of no more than 1 percent for incontinence and around 4 percent for impotence generally indicates a great deal of skill and experience.

The Nerve-Sparing Technique

The nerve-sparing technique allows the majority of patients to retain their sexual activities. The objective of using this technique is primarily to remove all of the cancer cells and secondly to preserve one or both of the bundles of nerves and blood vessels that are essential to having an erection.

In 1991, Dr. Patrick C. Walsh wrote an encouraging report in which he analyzed the postoperative sexual function in 503 men who had the operation that preserved or removed the neurovascular bundle(s) of their prostate. The procedure left both nerves intact; 90 percent of men under the age of fifty retained potency. Among those aged fifty to fifty-nine years old, 82 percent retained potency. For those aged sixty to sixty-nine years, 69 percent retained potency, and among those aged seventy and over, 22 percent did.

Moreover, every patient under age fifty with one nerve partially excised retained his potency. In the fifty to fifty-nine years of age group, 73 percent retained potency. For those aged sixty to sixty-nine, 50 percent did, and of those seventy and over, half did.

Results when one nerve was widely excised were only a little less encouraging, at least for patients under age fifty. Ninety-one percent of them retained potency. That rate fell to 58 percent for patients between ages fifty to fifty-nine; of those aged sixty-five to sixty-nine (the oldest in the study group), 47 percent retained potency.

CAUTIONS AND CONCERNS REGARDING SURGERY

Even if the nerves are spared, it may take many months or even a year or more to gradually regain the ability to have an erection. For example, if only one side of the nerves was saved, then the odds are still very low that you will regain your potency. Unfortunately, if the nerves are injured, they are very slow to heal.

Doctors should inform but not overly alarm the patient. This is not always easy to do. Certainly most men would prefer to go for the operation if it comes down to a choice between a sexually active life or no life at all.

... AND SOME COMFORT

After prostate removal to treat cancer, men who have no symptoms after six years will probably be free of cancer for the rest of their lives. So states a study from Baylor College of Medicine in Houston, where 436 men had their prostates removed to treat a cancer that had not spread to other parts of the body. Seventy of the patients had a recurrence of the cancer, but no new cases were reported after six years. Dr. Ozdal Dillioglugil, who led the research, comments that a hazard rate that falls steadily to zero suggests that the cancer was completely eradicated. The results support the effectiveness of radical prostatectomy in the treatment of prostate cancer.

CHAPTER TEN

Nonsurgical Treatments

John E. Weinberg, a leading researcher at the Dartmouth Medical School, distilled the proper approach to medical treatment: "It is inappropriate for the physician to prescribe the right treatment. It is appropriate for the patient to choose it."

Those words apply to all illnesses, including those of the prostate, and they underscore the importance of researching the available options in confronting an illness. This chapter looks at alternatives to surgery for prostate patients with prostate cancer.

TREATMENT OPTIONS

The patient should expect to be under the care of a competent urologist who will guide the patient in making the right choice. Hopefully, the urologist will make suggestions in a sensitive and confident manner, as the patient's mental attitude in dealing with this disease has considerable impact on the outcome.

Patients often assume that the doctor has all the answers and knows what type of treatment is best for the individual. The patient should discuss openly with his doctor all aspects of the numerous options, including goals, effects, and costs. It would be wise to have a partner and even other members of the family attend this discussion. Prostate cancer is a family disease—all members of the family will be impacted while the patient goes for treatment.

When prostate cancer is diagnosed, deciding on the type of treatment is not an easy choice. Let's explore the pros and cons of some of the options available.

Radiation Therapy

Radiation therapy involves the use of high-energy rays aimed at a specific area of the body to bombard and kill cancer cells. Most malignant cells are less able to repair radiation damage than normal cells.

A big advantage of radiation therapy is that it can be done on an outpatient basis, which is less costly than hospitalization. Each treatment takes about five to fifteen minutes, and the patient comes in for treatment five days a week for six to seven weeks.

By extending the period of time, the doses of radiation can remain small. This helps to prevent any adverse side effects to the rectum or bladder. It is also more effective in killing the cancer cells gradually over a period of time. Once the treatment is finished, no radioactivity remains.

Some doctors question whether this procedure actually kills the cells or just inhibits them from continuing their destruction. But most patients feel that if radiation therapy can allow them to live out their normal life span without symptoms, it is worthwhile.

One major disadvantage of radiation therapy is that the lymph nodes cannot be evaluated to see if the treatment is the correct one. It does not make sense to undergo this form of treatment and be subjected to the expense and discomfort unless the nodes can be identified to reasonably assure that the patient will benefit. The patient will have to be monitored via PSA tests to see if the cancer becomes active again.

Radiation therapy can also cause bladder, stomach, and intestinal discomfort, but this will usually go away. One unfounded fear is that it will cause the patient to go bald. If he does lose a little hair, it will be in the pubic area, where the beams of radiation are directed.

There is the danger that some of the rays may miss their intended target and damage healthy cells nearby. However, the healthy cells are better able to recover if the doses of radiation are small and are spread out over time. Radiation treatment may cause erectile dysfunction and impotence in approximately 25 to 50 percent of patients, but there is less than a 5 percent danger of incontinence.

Interstitial Radiotherapy or Brachytherapy

A century ago, Alexander Graham Bell described how a tiny fragment of radium sealed in a glass tube was inserted into a cancerous tumor to kill the tumor.

This early form of radiation therapy, now called interstitial radiotherapy or brachytherapy, has been developed to a point where urologists are impressed with its effectiveness compared to surgery for the treatment of prostate cancer.

For this treatment, the urologist refers the patient to a radiation oncologist—a cancer specialist who uses doses of radiation called "seeds," which are tiny pieces of radioactive material that are implanted permanently or temporarily by needle. Disc-sized capsules of radioactive palladium 103 or iodine 125 are placed inside the prostate to kill adjacent cancer cells. They are usually inserted through the skin directly into the prostate using the perineal approach (through the perineum).

Brachytherapy is done under anesthesia, and it takes about two hours. At considerably less cost than a total prostatectomy, it can be done on an outpatient basis. Usually, there is minor pain, and soreness or discomfort may last for around ten days.

About forty-five seeds are typically used, which are active for three to six months. They are then cast off and digested by the body. They do not emit any radiation outside the tumor that could cause any damage, but they do irradiate both malignant cells and healthy ones. The theory is that the healthy cells will heal while the cancerous ones should not.

As for side effects, brachytherapy carries less chance of difficulty in controlling urination than does surgery. The impotence rate is estimated at around 25 percent.

Dr. Heyoung McBride and Dr. William Homaday, staff members at Iowa Methodist John Stoddard Center, say the procedure has opened a new option for many of their patients. One advantage they cite is that the accuracy allows the seeds to deliver doses of radiation up to three times that of standard radiation, which at those doses would likely damage surrounding organs.

Another proponent of its use is Dr. John Koval, a radiation oncologist who comments that the radiation from the palladium does not spread very far. In fact, one centimeter (four-tenths of an inch) from the seed, the radiation level drops off dramatically, minimizing the effect on neighboring tissue and organs. Dr. Koval further comments that brachytherapy is preferred for those who have early stages of prostate cancer. For those with more advanced stages of the disease, it may be used in conjunction with other types of treatment.

The use of seed implants was initiated at Seattle's Northwest Hospital in 1986. More than 700 physicians around the world were trained in the procedure. They first used only iodine pellets. Soon afterward, a new seed called TheraSeed palladium 103 was introduced, offering a more aggressive attack on tumor cells than the iodine seed. Although longer-term studies are still desirable, the treatment has several advantages over invasive surgery for local tumors. As a one-time outpatient procedure, it's very cost-effective—half of what a radical prostatectomy would cost.

"I hesitate to endorse radioactive seed implantation for men who are good candidates for surgery, simply because there are no results documenting efficiency beyond five years. More research has to be done," counters the University of Michigan Medical School in Ann Arbor's Dr. Joseph E. Oesterling.

Still, the Pacific Northwest Cancer Foundation in 1995 reported a 91 percent success rate in controlling early-onset prostate cancer with seed implantation therapy. In another study, 188 patients with more aggressive prostate cancer were treated with both external-beam radiation therapy and seed implantation. The six-year results show a 78 percent disease-free success rate from prostatic carcinoma.

Bladder and bowel irritation are substantially reduced with the implants compared to external-beam radiation, even though the implants deliver about twice as much radiation to the prostate, according to Dr. Michael Dattoli, a radiation oncologist at University Community Hospital in Tampa, Florida. He has found that incontinence rarely occurs, and impotence occurs in about 5 to 10 percent of men under the age of seventy, similar to external radiation and much better than surgery.

Implanting palladium 103, which is more expensive than iodine 125, costs between $5,000 and $11,000 depending on the size of the prostate, Dr. Dattoli said. Surgery, by comparison, costs between $20,000 and $28,000, excluding the recovery period at home.

However, brachytherapy is not for everyone. A disadvantage is cited for patients who had a TURP, as it can make the process less effective or increase the complication rate. The TURP changes the geography of the prostate gland and may interfere with uniform placement of seeds. In one study of 274 prostate cancer patients with brachytherapy at the Northwest Tumor Institute, a forty-month follow-up found incontinence in fourteen of 274 patients. A closer look shows that ninety of these 274 patients had a prior TURP, including all fourteen of those with incontinence. In the other 184 patients without TURPs, none had developed incontinence.

According to Dr. Kent Wallner, a radiation oncologist at Memorial Sloan-Kettering Cancer Center in New York, brachytherapy is not ideal for patients with larger tumors or those whose cancer has spread beyond the prostate capsule. For these patients, external-beam radiation continues to be the treatment of choice. He said that the procedure appears to be most effective for small, localized tumors at stages A1, A2, B1, and B2.

There are side effects, the most common of which is irritation of the urinary tract—a sudden urgency to urinate, burning or irritation, or blood in the urine. The same symptoms may show up during a bowel movement. Problems of infection of the prostate may also develop.

Hormone Therapy

Hormone therapy is used mainly for metastatic and recurring prostate cancers that cause bone pain and bladder obstruction. This type of therapy works better if it is started as early as possible after the cancer has reached an advanced stage.

The main objective of this therapy is to lower the level of male hormones.

The spread of prostate cancer is fueled by testosterone, a male hormone produced by the male testicles; therefore, a treatment that deprives the cancer cell of testosterone can slow the growth of prostate cancer. The disadvantages of hormone therapy are that it can cause water retention, breast growth and tenderness, hot flashes, and symptoms such as stomach upset, nausea, and vomiting. Although hormone therapy will not cause a patient to speak in a high pitch or make him look feminine, it may lower his sexual appetite or impair his ability to have an erection. The treatment for some men works very well and they may go many years with no evidence of cancer growth. Some will have substantial cancer shrinkage and regression, while others may have favorable results for only a short period of time.

This process has advanced little in the past twenty years. Hormone therapy is an effective means in some cases, but it is not a cure.

LHRH Therapy

LHRH therapy consists of giving the patient a drug called luteinizing hormone-releasing hormone analogue, or LHRH analogue.

The drug is basically a copy of a natural hormone in the body that stimulates the production of testosterone. LHRH therapy is a simple method, involving an injection once a month. The injection stimulates a burst of testosterone for approximately fourteen days. The patient's body reacts to this as if it is producing too much testosterone. It closes down its hormone production, resulting in a level drop to almost zero (a similar result occurs if the testicles are removed). To maintain this level, the patient has to continue the injections.

LHRH therapy is as effective as an orchiectomy (removal of the testicles), but it does not require surgery. It also avoids the side effects of estrogen therapy. It does, however, often cause impotence and a loss of sexual desire in about half of all patients.

Other disadvantages of LHRH therapy are that monthly office visits are required and, in a small percentage of patients, the therapy may cause a brief increase of cancer symptoms, such as bone pain, before the testosterone level begins to fall. The therapy consists of a large needle inserted deep into the muscle, and it should be administered by a doctor or a nurse. It is also very expensive, costing about $8,500 a year, but this is usually covered by Medicare.

Cryosurgery

In cryosurgery, a metal probe is placed directly into the tumor tissue, and the tumor is destroyed by freezing. This is accomplished by liquid oxygen that is circulated through the probes, freezing the tissue of the prostate. The process is monitored by ultrasound. This procedure takes just two or three hours under spinal or general anesthesia; patients report little pain and are able to resume normal activities within a week. The process works best when the prostate gland weighs 40 grams or less and has never been operated on. A 1993 *Cancer Communication Newsletter* favorably compared cryosurgery to radical prostatectomy. The article listed the advantages of cryosurgery as follows:

- No surgical incision is required. Usually an overnight hospital stay is not necessary, and in some cases it can be performed on an outpatient basis.
- No blood needs to be taken for autologous transfusion (using the patient's blood for transfusion during surgery).
- Usually only one day of recovery is needed before resuming normal activity.
- Incontinence and impotence occur much less frequently than with a radical prostatectomy.
- It is considerably less expensive than a radical prostatectomy.
- If necessary, it can be repeated if residual cancerous tissue is found.

However, proof of the procedure's efficacy is lacking. Only about 115 men have undergone cryosurgery over the last fifteen months at the only hospitals to use the procedure so far, Allegheny General Hospital in Pittsburgh and M. D. Anderson Cancer Center in Houston. There have been no published follow-up studies, and such short-term results wouldn't mean much even if they did exist—if the cancer isn't completely eliminated, it can reappear in ten or fifteen years.

There are concerns that some of the malignant cells may not be frozen and that cells outside the process will escape being treated. Other disadvantages are that it can be very irritating to the bladder and urethra. Although only temporary, about 50 percent of the patients complain of some degree of swelling in the penile and scrotal area. Others complain of frequent urination without any warning, blood in their urine, a burning pain when urinating, impotence, and discomfort in the rectal wall.

At this point, medical opinions of cryosurgery vary widely, and further research will be needed in order to determine its long-term value.

Chemotherapy

Chemotherapy involves the use of powerful drugs to kill cancer cells. The drugs circulate throughout the body in the bloodstream and kill any rapidly growing cells, including healthy ones. To destroy cancer cells while minimizing the harm to healthy ones, the drugs are carefully controlled in dosage and frequency.

There are many different chemotherapy drugs, each with its own strengths and weaknesses. Often the drugs are used in combination.

Since the chemotherapy drugs circulate throughout the body and affect healthy as well as cancerous cells, they produce many side effects. These include hair loss, nausea, fatigue, pain, vomiting, diarrhea, reduced ability of the blood to clot, and an increased risk of infection. Most of the side effects disappear when the treatment is stopped.

The use of chemotherapy in treating prostate cancer is largely limited to stage D, when the cancer has spread to other parts of the body. Chemotherapy drugs do not work well in many men with prostate cancer, and therefore they are rarely recommended as routine treatment. If all else fails with other treatments, chemotherapy will be used to slow the growth of the disease.

Chemotherapy is more commonly used to treat other types of cancers by stopping or slowing their growth and relieving the symptoms. Cancers that have been successfully "cured" with chemotherapy include testicular cancers, certain leukemias, and lymphomas.

One problem of using conventional chemotherapy methods to treat prostate cancer is that patients are usually elderly and have other medical problems and are therefore unable to tolerate chemotherapy in efficient doses. Chemotherapeutic drugs, conventionally administered, are most successfully used in patients who are younger and healthy.

One major problem inherent in chemotherapy is that many of the highly potent drugs used do not reach the bloodstream effectively.

With more research and development in this area, it is possible that more workable drugs will be developed.

One newer technique on the horizon is implantable chemotherapy. Dr. Perinchery Narayan, Associate Professor of Urology and Specialist in Oncology at the University of California Medical Center in San Francisco, says that this technique "may represent new hope for patients with recurrence of prostate cancer."

Dr. Narayan and his colleagues implant a chemotherapeutic drug, suspended in collagen matrix, near the cancer. This method allows the drug to be given in smaller doses than by a conventional route (intravenously or intra-arterially), while the concentration achieved in the area of the cancer is higher.

Since the chemotherapeutic drug doesn't flow through the rest of the body, the toxicity to the system is minimal. The technique is especially practical for older patients, who are at higher risk for complications from surgery.

Chemotherapy is often used in treating malignant growths but is not as popular a choice for most oncologists in treating prostate cancer. The side effects may outweigh the benefits the patient will derive from the treatments. Hopefully, a drug will be discovered that will slow the cancerous growth without causing the emotional and physical side effects.

PART IV

Surgery

CHAPTER ELEVEN

From the Waiting Room to the Recovery Room

The decision to have surgery can be reached by a number of routes:

- A BPH patient's prostate may have continued its growth; his symptoms, instead of diminishing, may have increased to the point of intolerability. According to Dr. Steven Gumbert, cancer of the prostate occurs more frequently in men with benign prostatic hyperplasia—although hyperplasia has not been shown to actually be the cause.
- The patient may be legitimately concerned that his cancer tests have produced "false negative" results. This means that he may have an inaccurate test result that fails to show the presence of a cancerous tumor, which can later be found by a biopsy or other medical diagnosis. He may be concerned about the possibility that a cancerous prostate nodule is lurking undiscovered, ready to spread to other parts of the body.
- The patient may be diagnosed with prostate cancer, and he and his doctor may have determined that nonsurgical options such as radiation and hormone treatment (see Chapter 10, "Prostate Cancer: Nonsurgical Treatments") are unlikely to resolve the problem.

If you (together with your doctor and your family) have made the decision to have surgery, then you will need to make preparations for the time before and after the operation. This chapter will cover the important factors in planning for surgery.

SELECTING A HOSPITAL

Many hospitals are available for surgical procedures on the prostate. It is a very competitive business out there. But which one should you select? This is a most important consideration.

Several years ago, a subcommittee of the U.S. House of Representatives reported on the surgical performance of American doctors. It concluded that an individual may have twice the chance of dying from an operation simply by having the procedure performed at one hospital rather than another. While it's not clear whether that troubling statistic impugns the doctors who performed the operations or the hospitals where they took place (or something else entirely), it should provide additional motivation to check out both.

Over thirty million Americans were admitted to hospitals last year. Yet probably only a handful of patients were aware of the difference in ratings of the many institutions. Do your homework and check out these ratings. Full-length guides are available in bookstores, or you can contact any of the following groups:

- Consumers' Guide to Hospitals, 733 15th Street NW, Suite 820, Washington, D.C. 20005.
- American Hospital Association, 325 Seventh Street W, Washington, D.C. 20004, or call (202) 638-1100; ask for the free brochure "Helping You Choose a Hospital."
- The Joint Commission on Accreditation of Healthcare Organizations, (708) 916-5800. It offers a free brochure, "Helping You Choose...Quality of Hospital Care," and sells performance reports on selected hospitals for $30 each.

THE PATIENT'S BILL OF RIGHTS

The American Hospital Association has prepared a Patient's Bill of Rights with the expectation that observance of these rights will help provide improved care for the patient by the physician and the hospital. It should be posted at the admissions desk of every hospital. You may want to ask if the hospital adheres to the voluntary code.

The Patient's Bill of Rights maintains that a personal relationship between the doctor and the patient is essential to providing proper medical care. There are twelve provisions in this Bill of Rights, which I have paraphrased below:

1. Proper and respectful medical care is a fundamental right of every patient.
2. Patients have the right to review their medical charts and to ask their doctor for a copy of all their medical records. If the patient can't understand the information, then it should be given to someone else on his or her behalf.
3. The doctor has no right to treat you without your "informed consent." (Unfortunately, this provision is not practiced by many doctors.)
4. A patient has the right to not accept the recommendation of a doctor, but the doctor has a right to inform the patient of the consequences of not accepting his or her recommendation.
5. The release of patient records without his or her consent is forbidden.
6. This provision expands on Provision 5, further specifying "all communications."
7. The hospital must be prompt in responding to a patient's request for services. Also, the hospital cannot transfer the patient to another hospital without giving reasons for the transfer.

8. The patient has the right to obtain information about the relationship of the hospital with other institutions or corporations, if related to his or her medical case.

9. No hospital may use the patient in experimentation without his or her consent.

10. The patient has a right to continuous care, either in the hospital or at home. In essence, the patient's physician or a delegate must be on call.

11. The patient has to receive an adequate explanation pertaining to medical charges.

12. The patient has the right to review a hospital's code of conduct for the patient, which details what is expected of the patient and should be posted on the wall of the admittance office.

MEDICAL COSTS AND INSURANCE PROCEDURES

To avoid as much stress as possible, it would be wise to look into medical costs before going into the hospital. You certainly don't want to be asked questions about your insurance and how the medical expenses will be handled the day of your admittance without having this information readily available.

Most people have some type of medical coverage, but few understand what they have. This may be the first time you have reviewed the benefits since you received your policy, and you may not remember or understand what the benefits are. Rather than agonize over trying to interpret insurance lingo, call your agent for help. Clarify the amount of your deductible, the daily hospital benefit, and so on.

When you register at the hospital, have your identification card and all forms ready. The last thing you want to be bothered with is having to obtain additional information at the last minute. If you have disability coverage, get that paperwork started as soon as possible.

Medicare

Most prostate surgery patients are senior citizens, so a familiarity with Medicare is important. Medicare is a federal health insurance program for Americans who are sixty-five years of age and older or who are disabled.

Medicare comes in two parts: hospital insurance and medical insurance. Most people have both parts. Hospital insurance, sometimes called Part A, covers inpatient hospital care and certain follow-up care. You have paid for it through your Social Security taxes. Medical insurance, sometimes called Part B, pays for physicians' services and some other services not covered by hospital insurance. Medical insurance is optional, and a moderate premium is charged. Unless you decline medical insurance protection, the premium will be automatically deducted from your Social Security benefit.

If you applied for retirement or survivor's benefits before your sixty-fifth birthday, you do not need to file a separate application for Medicare. Your coverage starts automatically at age sixty-five, even if you have not yet received your Medicare card in the mail. You will receive information in the mail before you turn sixty-five that will explain what you need to do, or you can call 800-772-1213 for information.

THE HOSPITAL STAY

You should plan to make your stay in the hospital as pleasant as possible. Relatives and friends with a good sense of humor should be encouraged to visit, since laughter helps reduce stress. Medical research now suggests that laughter gives a workout to bodily organs and triggers the secretion of endorphins in the brain, which fosters a sense of relaxation and well-being and dulls the perception of pain.

Dr. William Fry, a psychiatrist affiliated with Stanford University and a student of laughter for three decades, says that laughing one hundred times a day is equivalent to about ten minutes of rowing. As Dr. Marvin Eitterring of the New Jersey School of Osteopathic Medicine puts it, the thorax, heart, lungs, diaphragm, abdomen, and liver are given a massage during a hearty laugh. (I have often thought that laughter had something to do with the longevity of famous comedians such as Eddie Cantor, Jack Benny, Myron Cohen, George Jessel, Bob Hope, and George Burns.)

Consider taking along a tape recorder with headphones so that you can listen to comedy tapes while in the hospital. Listening to classical music may also be beneficial and help you to adjust to the inevitable pain and loneliness. Be sure to take along your favorite bathrobe, pictures of your family, and anything that will put you in a positive frame of mind.

Meditation, biofeedback, and any exercise you can do to put your mind at ease are all helpful. Many books are available that explain how to use these techniques. They underscore the importance of visualization in controlling a disease and maintaining health. The visualization methods used by Dr. O. Carl Simonton with cancer patients demonstrate that an individual's will can play a major part in the course of any disease. *The Will to Live*, a book by A. J. Hutschnecker, is also very helpful.

TALK WITH YOUR DOCTOR

Have your urologist talk you through what you can expect to happen from day one when you enter the hospital until your discharge date, including your medication, the type of anesthesia that will be given, the nature of the surgery, the type of pain to be expected, what complications might develop, the length of your stay, and anything else that will help you avoid unnecessary surprises. I suggest that you have a close friend or relative present for this conference so they will be better prepared to help you through this difficult period.

Your doctor should discuss with you the various procedures that will take place, especially the many tubes that will be inserted into your body. If you have an aversion to pills, you should discuss your preference for as small a dosage as possible to relieve pain.

Above all, it is important to think positively and realize how fortunate you are to be placed in a modern facility with an experienced surgeon and a competent support staff. The chances of a speedy and complete recovery are excellent.

PREPARATION FOR SURGERY

You will probably enter the hospital the day before surgery or the day of surgery. Routine blood and urine tests will be taken. A chest X-ray and electrocardiogram may be ordered. Some tests may not be needed if they were taken prior to entering the hospital.

Some urologists will recommend that you have two to three pints of your blood stored in the event that you require a transfusion during the operation. In light of the possibility that you could contract hepatitis or AIDS if blood from someone else is used, it certainly is something that you should do. It is not at all painful—it is slightly inconvenient, as you will have to have blood drawn one pint at a time—but it is well worth the time, effort, and expense.

Your pubic area will be shaved in order to help prevent infection. You will probably be advised not to eat or drink after midnight.

You also will be visited by your anesthesiologist, who will discuss the type of anesthesia that will be used. Prior to the surgery, a mild sedative will be given to relax you and to make the anesthetic more pleasant for you.

DURING SURGERY

Now on to the operating room, where the anesthesia is given and the operation begins. You will probably be given a general anesthesia, which will put you completely to sleep. Sleep is induced by a fast-acting barbiturate such as sodium pentothal given intravenously, after which you will be kept asleep by an inhalant anesthetic agent. The other option is spinal anesthesia, with which you are awake but the lower part of your body has no feeling. These two methods are usually not accompanied by the postoperative nausea and vomiting so common in the past when ether and similar anesthetic agents were used. Most importantly, they provide a greater margin of safety.

During the surgery and for a brief period afterward, an intravenous tube will provide you with nutrition and medication. Your blood pressure, pulse, and breathing will be monitored carefully by specially trained nurses. During the surgery, a Foley catheter is inserted into your bladder, which serves two functions: to drain the bladder while healing takes place and to act as a splint around the area where the bladder neck was stitched so the stump of the urethra can heal. If you had an epidural (skin-deep) anesthetic, a small catheter will be left in place for several days to provide a steady or intermittent drip of a pain-relieving solution.

AFTER THE OPERATION

After the operation, the Foley catheter will remain in the penis opening. This special catheter, which has a water-filled balloon on the bladder end to keep it in place continuously, drains the urine into a sterile collection bag (see page 77). It is usually left in for two to four days after a TURP and for up to a week after open surgery. It may cause bladder spasms or make you feel that you have to relieve yourself. The nurse can give you pain pills or other medication to help. When I had surgery for BPH, the severe pain of bladder spasms was the most difficult part of my hospital stay.

If you have suprapubic surgery, you will have an additional catheter to provide better urine drainage for the first few days after the operation

Recovery

After the operation, you will be placed on a special postoperative cart and moved to the recovery room, where nurses with special training in this area will check your blood pressure and pulse, observe how the catheter is draining, and monitor your breathing. If you need a sedative, your urologist will be close by.

When everything stabilizes, you will be ready to go to your room, where your relatives can visit you.

A nurse will probably have to assist you during recovery, as you could very well be a little dizzy and unsteady as you try to get in and out of bed. The support you receive from the nurses is very important during the recovery process. A recent study shows that nursing care is vitally important, not only in providing comfort but in preventing and managing possible complications.

The nurse will advise you on how to adjust to the catheter and how to keep it clean. You will still have it in you when you are discharged, and it will later be removed. If you have blood clots after the surgery, your catheter will be irrigated frequently. This causes some discomfort, but it is necessary to keep the flow going. The urine may look pink until irrigation is stopped, when it turns darker red. It will clear up by the time you are released from the hospital.

During most of your stay in the hospital, you will continue receiving fluids through your veins with an IV. Your IV tube will be removed as soon as you can eat and drink again to the satisfaction of your doctor. You will be advised to drink plenty of liquids; eight cups a day are recommended to help flush the bladder. Stool softeners are often given so that you won't have to strain when you have a bowel movement.

Your stitches will be removed about a week after the surgery. Fortunately, removing the stitches is not a painful procedure.

Postoperative Urination Remember not to expect miracles. You still may not urinate normally after the catheter is taken out. You also may feel a painful or burning sensation. A common sensation is the urge to urinate frequently and difficulty in controlling your urine flow—almost a flashback to the reasons for having the surgery, but this will pass (no pun intended). It may take a few days or even months before you get back to a normal urination frequency.

One unpleasant aspect of recovery is the discomfort associated with the operation. Even with medication, you will experience some pain. Especially aggravating are the bladder spasms. They are your bladder's way of telling you that it doesn't like the irritation caused by the catheter. It tries to get rid of the foreign object by squeezing down on the bladder, causing a very painful cramping in the lower abdominal area. It comes without warning and will last a minute or more, but it will certainly spoil your day.

It helps if you close your eyes and picture yourself in a pleasant environment, perhaps at the ocean or mountains, and say to yourself, "It is only a matter of time and this will be behind me."

Postoperative Walking A day after the surgery, your doctor will probably ask you to walk around the hospital to prevent blood clots and pneumonia. Walking through the hospital ward will break up the monotony of the hospital stay and contribute to your rehabilitation. This exercise is also important to stimulate normal bowel movements. You are, of course, not ready to jump out of bed and go walking briskly around the hospital. At this stage, you should move very slowly. You will notice that you don't have the energy that you had prior to surgery, and you may feel tired or even lightheaded and dizzy. If so, don't fight it; lie down and, if necessary, ask for help.

Start walking slowly and try to extend the duration of the walk each day. Be sure not to overdo it, as frequency is more important than mileage at this stage. If you happen to walk past a full-length mirror on your daily excursion, you may be surprised at the image of yourself with all the tubes connected and exclaim, "I look like the bionic man!"

GOING HOME

After four or five days, or perhaps even sooner, you will be ready to go home. A major reason to go home as soon as possible is that hospitals, no matter how highly they are rated, are potentially a source of dangerous and complicated forms of infection. You will probably be placed on a wheelchair and wheeled to the hospital pickup site, where your relative or friend will take you home. This can be a most pleasant journey, as you reflect on the fact that you have finally parted company with the obstructive tissue that has caused you so much grief.

Now the body has to adjust and heal. It could take six to eight weeks for the urine to flow in an orderly manner. For some who have had problems for a long time prior to the operation, it may be months before the bladder returns to normal. You should avoid high-fat foods and eat a balanced diet including fruits and vegetables every day. Foods that are rich in bulk and fiber will help you to avoid constipation; bleeding can be caused by straining to have a bowel movement. A proper diet could also help to prevent a recurrence of malignant cells.

Exercise

Continue your exercise, gradually increasing the level and pace of walking that you did while in the hospital. Be sure not to overdo it.

You will probably be advised by your doctor to not get on a bicycle until several weeks after you have had surgery. It is not wise to put pressure on your perineum (the area of your body between the scrotum and anus), as this was the site of the surgery. If you are a cycling enthusiast, you will have plenty of time to resume this activity later. You may want to add padding and get a wider seat on your bicycle to assist the rehabilitation process and prevent pain.

You should wait several weeks before playing tennis, to avoid any sudden strain on the body. You can certainly go out and hit balls at a relaxed pace, but avoid any competitive matches and stay away from the "A" players.

Golf should also be resumed at a leisurely pace. The early stages of your recovery may be the one time when you should use a golf cart instead of walking the course.

Wait until you are fully recovered before you resume jogging or using a treadmill, step machine, or other exercise equipment. Your doctor can help you to assess when you are ready. Each individual recovers at a different rate, depending to a great extent on what kind of condition you were in prior to the surgery.

Light swimming should be all right as soon as the catheter comes out and the incision is healed. Working in your garden and doing light housework should also be fine.

You should not do the shopping for at least ten days to two weeks. Avoid driving, since the incision is still healing and tender; suddenly applying the brakes could tear the incision open.

Your doctor can advise you about when to resume sexual activity. It is very important to listen, as you could tear open the incision.

It is most important not to return to work or other normal activities without your doctor's blessing. You may feel impatient, but you do not want to create problems that will require additional surgery. Your return to employment will depend on the type of work you do and how quickly your energy level is restored. If you work at a desk or you have an occupation that requires a minimum of physical activity, you may be ready three to four weeks after the surgery. If your work requires a lot of physical exertion, returning to it will take longer. Your body will let you know. You do not want to sit down in front of the TV all day. You will recuperate best by being active without overdoing it.

FOLLOW-UP AND MONITORING

Now it is up to you, more than your doctor or anyone else, to maintain and protect your health. Keep your appointments for postoperative checkups. During recovery, if you experience excessive pain or bleeding, do not hesitate to call your doctor.

Many urologists will agree that surgery offers the best long-term survival for the patient. With a high level of confidence, a patient can look forward to a life free of any more need of surgery or radical treatment. Unfortunately, however, after all you and your family have been through, there is the possibility that cancerous cells could still develop. The growth of cancer may be more dependent on the inherent tumor biology than on the particular type of treatment.

Needless to say, you do not want to even think about the possibility that cancerous cells could develop. But since the possibility exists, the doctor will want to continue examining and monitoring you to determine if the disease did recur or if possibly some cancer was not taken out.

Remember, though, that you have received medical treatment that probably surpasses any care you could have received in any other country. If you develop problems following surgery, keep in mind that your chances of living out a full and healthy life are excellent. Hippocrates once said, "Be thy own physician." There is a lot you can do to support the activities of your urologist. Develop a positive attitude—your brain sends messages to all parts of your body. Concentrate on the good. After all, you made it. You are the same person that you were prior to having the episode with the prostate cancer. Later chapters will provide more information on how to enrich the quality of your life.

CHAPTER TWELVE

Coping with Complications

Ask any male what he fears most about having surgery in the area of his sexual organs and, if he's honest, he will probably tell you that he fears becoming impotent or incontinent. Often, such fears will result in delaying treatment for prostate problems. Such resistance can create further problems for a patient with an enlarged prostate, but if he has prostate cancer, this resistance may be a matter of life or death.

It is not easy for a surgeon to avoid causing some damage, especially when performing a radical prostatectomy. In this operation, the surgeon removes the entire prostate gland and the seminal vesicles. The part of the urethra that passes through the prostate is also removed. Sometimes it is difficult for the surgeon to eliminate all the cancer without causing the permanent loss of bladder control and erectile dysfunction.

The nerves that control urinary and sexual functions are extremely small and are located near the prostate gland. To be sure to get all the cancer, the surgeon may have to cut the nerves as well as the sphincter muscle, and damage can result. The main priority of the surgery is to get out all the cancer cells and not leave any behind. The next priority is to preserve potency. The chances of achieving both objectives are steadily improving through the nerve-sparing technique (see Chapter 9).

Despite the advances in surgical techniques, however, some complications may develop after an operation on the prostate. This chapter will cover possible problems and how to deal with them, and it will also discuss the latest treatments and drugs.

IMPOTENCE

The thought of losing the ability to have an erection is undoubtedly why many males opt for the watchful waiting option. Although the possibility of becoming impotent does exist following surgery, doctors should inform the patient that the nerve-sparing technique, developed in the last several years, protects the nerves necessary to get an erection.

Dr. Patrick C. Walsh has had excellent results in using the nerve-sparing technique. In an update of an evaluation of 600 men who have had his nerve-sparing operation from one and a half to eight years previously, the local recurrence rate at five years was 4 percent, distant metastases (cancer that had spread to other organs or tissues through the lymphatic or blood systems) was 7 percent; and 3 percent died of the disease. Ten-year to fifteen-year evaluations are planned.

Fears about impotence are not totally unreasonable; even with nerve-sparing surgical techniques, the nerves may be damaged. If the nerves have been saved, it still may still take many months after prostate surgery, or even a year to two, before a man can again have an erection. Unfortunately, nerves take a long time to heal. Young men in good overall health are apt to have less problems with the return of erections. Psychological, emotional, and personal belief factors play an important role in the ability to regain potency.

Surgery isn't the only treatment that can create sexual problems. A variety of methods, such as hormone therapy, cryosurgery, radiation, and others, can affect the ability to have and sustain an erection. Watching and waiting can also cause impotency—the cancer can spread and grow through the prostate, damaging the nerves. Also, fear, anxiety, and stress can inhibit a man from having an erection. But if it's a choice between life or sex, wouldn't life win over sex? In most cases, though it may take a while after the treatment, sooner or later the penis will rise to the occasion.

If erectile dysfunction does develop following an operation, much can be done to alleviate the problem. The urologist can advise the patient of the treatments that are available. Since the costs and inconvenience of treating impotence can be considerable, the patient may want to seek counsel from a sexual therapist before trying the various methods that are available to overcome erectile problems. With his partner, he should experiment with various ways to satisfy each other. The man can still have orgasms. The orgasms will be dry, because the prostate no longer produces fluid, but this doesn't mean an absence of sexual pleasure.

A patient recovering from surgery should also give his body a chance to adjust to the operation to see if help is actually needed. It may take many months to determine if impotence is permanent. Unfortunately, many patients look for an immediate, simple solution to their sexual inactivity. They purchase exotic products that promise to restore their potency and even make them into sexual giants. These products are usually worthless (except perhaps as a psychological boost), and they could be dangerous. Laetrile is a good example of misguided hopes leading desperate people to place their lives in danger.

Some products selling the promise of enhanced sexual vitality contain ground-up animal parts and are therefore perilous to the African rhinoceros and other animals. Fortunately for these animals, the FDA has banned the aphrodisiacs from being sold, as they do not measure up to their claims.

There are legitimate ways to alleviate this common difficulty. If the patient has posttreatment impotence, he should discuss it openly with his doctor and mate. Medical professionals are available to help, and there are a variety of ways to enjoy sexual activity. If you have this problem, you are certainly not alone. For twenty million Americans, the problem of not being to able to achieve or maintain an erection is most serious. Contrary to what many doctors used to think, they now believe the cause is not psychological but biological. A variety of treatments are available to help with this problem.

Testosterone Treatment

In the past, men who had problems with impotence would go to their doctor's office for two or three weeks for a series of testosterone injections into the buttocks or thigh, or they would wear a testosterone patch.

Today, a patch has become available that appears to be very promising. In a recent study, impotent men had two androderm patches applied nightly on the abdomen, back, or upper arms. Ninety-two percent of the participants found that their testosterone levels were steadily boosted and that they could achieve and maintain erection. The only complaint was irritation of the skin where the patches were applied. It is also an expensive process: a month's worth of daily treatments costs more than $72 wholesale.

There is another type of patch called Testoderm, which is produced by Alza. This one is applied to the scrotal skin, as this skin is thick with a rich blood supply and is unnoticeable. The testosterone passes from the patch through the skin and into the bloodstream. The main objective of the patch is to alleviate the deficiency of testosterone. A study in the late 1980s indicated that forty-five out of seventy-two men were able to increase their sexual activity and maintain normal levels. Hardly any reported any discomfort wearing the patch. A patient using this product should have his cholesterol level checked to make sure it is not radically affected, which has been a problem with this treatment.

Drug Therapy

Drugs may be used to help a man overcome impotence. In many cases, more testing is needed, and the treatments may be awkward or even painful, but many men will accept any drawbacks to regain their virility.

Papaverine This drug is injected directly into the side of the penis. It causes the arteries of the penis to dilate, increasing the flow of blood to the penis. It also causes less blood to leave. With this increased flow, many men will be able to achieve a firm erection.

Sildenafil This is another new drug that looks promising, but it needs more testing before it can be approved. It blocks an enzyme that can prevent erection by allowing blood to flow out of the erectile tissue. So far, researchers are very optimistic and they expect Sildenafil to come before the U.S. Food and Drug Administration (FDA) for review before 1997.

Prostaglandin This is another vein-dilating drug. It has recently received FDA approval under the trade name of Caverject. It is made by Upjohn, and some insurance companies may pay for its use as a prescription drug. After the drug is injected, the penis becomes rigid and is ready to perform within fifteen to twenty minutes. The erection can last for over an hour, which is something not commonly experienced by a man before surgery. A disadvantage is that the injection can cause bleeding, swelling, or bruising of the penis. It is sold in six-packs of injection kits. It comes in a vial with a sterile sponge in a disposable box and costs about $25 a dose.

Ginko biloba This is an herbal product that produces harder, stronger, longer-lasting erections and is considered one of the best by investigators in Germany who tested the product. In a recent study, twenty men who could only have erections when injecting special drugs into their penises were able to have spontaneous erections (without drugs) and experienced measurable increases in the hardness of the penis throughout its length. This was after nine months of taking a 50-milligram capsule of Ginko biloba three times a day.

VIP Researchers in Israel are awaiting approval for a cream they have developed that will help impotent men achieve an erection. They combined a chemical called vasoactive intestinal peptide (VIP) with stearic acid (a creamy substance) and applied it to the penises of castrated rats; as a result, the rats became sexually active. VIP has been around a long time and has been used as an injection treatment for impotence. This is the first time it has been applied in cream form to the penis. As with most physical medicine approaches, it works best for men suffering from a physical rather than psychological cause of impotence.

Vacuum Devices

Vacuum pumps work for almost every man whether his nerves are functioning or not. The penis is placed in a plastic cylinder, and a pump creates a vacuum inside the tube. The penis becomes erect, and a tension band is then slipped around the base of the penis to maintain the erection. The vacuum device is then removed.

The tension band can usually be kept on for as long as thirty minutes, and a man should generally be able to sustain the firmness until the sexual act is completed. It will not work to the satisfaction of everyone, but with the proper guidance it may be very fulfilling.

The main criticism of the vacuum pump is that it is unnatural to use a device for the sexual act, and many complain that the ring is uncomfortable to wear. The cost is under $500, and it does require a prescription.

Penile Implants

If all else fails, penile implants—also referred to as "prostheses"—are available to provide an erection. A new industry has sprung up to provide these devices, which are being advertised to have promising results. You should consult your urologist if you are considering purchasing one. They do require surgery, with its inherent risks and pain as well as considerable expense.

Penile implants come in four types: bendable, mechanical, inflatable with a pump, and inflatable without a pump.

The bendable is the easiest to use and is less likely to break, as it has almost no parts that can break or malfunction. It consists of silver wires that are braided inside a silicone sheath and then implanted in the penis. The penis will stay rigid, but the patient can bend it to tuck it in his pants or to urinate. When he desires to have intercourse, it can be bent into a straight position.

Mechanical implants consist of wire bound into a series of cups. These can be bent and are easier to maneuver than the bendable implants. The penis is always rigid, but it can be bent to conceal it or to urinate.

Inflatable implants that make use of pumps provide a more natural erection than the other products. A pump is placed in the scrotum between the testicles. When the pump is squeezed, it brings fluid into the pump cylinder, which slightly increases the diameter and length of the penis. To return the penis to its normal size, the release valve is squeezed. Often, however, technical problems develop that require additional surgery.

There are many inflatable implants that do not require pumps. They all have chambers of fluid. When the tip of the unit is squeezed, it brings fluid to the device, which causes it to increase the diameter of the penis. When the patient bends the implant, it activates the release valve and the penis reverts to its normal size.

A urologist can help with the decision of which type of implant to select and where to obtain it. It takes the incision about five weeks to heal before you can use the device. If you total up the surgery and hospitalization plus the purchase of the devices, the costs of penile implants can range from $2,000 to over $10,000 or more.

Before deciding to make a purchase, consider the fact that the problem of erectile dysfunction may be psychological. Sex counseling may be more appropriate to resolve the problem. The patient should discuss it openly with his mate and urologist before looking for other, expensive solutions.

PRIAPISM

One rare complication of surgery is a condition called priapism. This occurs when an erection develops and will not go away. This is a serious condition. If priapism occurs and lasts over an unusual period of time, the urologist should be called immediately, for it could result in permanent damage.

Medications for this condition are administered topically or with intraurethral suppositories. The urologist can advise the patient regarding these medications and whether they are suitable for the patient.

URINARY INCONTINENCE

Another possible complication of prostate surgery is incontinence. This condition afflicts twelve million Americans. Two percent to 5 percent of men undergoing prostate surgery suffer from severe or total incontinence. It is a most discomforting and humiliating problem; losing control of urination during exertion or a simple sneeze can cause shame.

Two mechanisms control male urinary continence; each has to work properly in order for a man to have voluntary control of urination. One mechanism is the musculature that surrounds much of the prostate gland and lies outside the true capsule of the prostate.

Its function is to maintain the tone of the urethra and the bladder neck and to keep them in a closed position except when the body is urinating. Severe damage to this area can lead to incontinence.

The other mechanism is the external urethral sphincter. If the surgeon damages this muscle during surgery, the result can be stress incontinence, which means an involuntary loss of urine when increased pressure develops within the abdomen and squeezes down on the bladder.

As with impotence, there are many ways to alleviate this condition. When an involuntary loss of urine persists beyond the period of hospitalization, various medications and treatments are available.

Collagen Injections

One popular treatment for incontinence is injections of collagen into tissue. Collagen is the protein extract of connective tissue from cattle. A recent investigation indicated that only 27 percent of men who received collagen injections were significantly helped by them. For some unknown reason, it is much more effective in women.

Collagen injections are easy to administer and typically do not cause any side effects, but this is an expensive procedure.

Kegel Exercises

Another technique used to treat incontinence is the Kegel exercise. This involves alternately tightening and relaxing the muscles of the floor of the pelvis to improve their tone and strength. The exercise is done throughout the day. You probably do this often without realizing it, for example when you are urinating and suddenly stop before you are through.

This exercise was developed by gynecologist Dr. Arnold Kegel for women who had trouble holding their urine after childbirth. Thousands of women and men have also increased their sexual responsiveness by doing this exercise. It is recommended by many therapists. Many males report stronger and more pleasurable orgasms as a result. It's also been helpful to men with erection problems and those who do not experience much feeling in their pelvic area.

Artificial Sphincter

Another technique to help the incontinent patient is the implantation of an artificial sphincter. This is not beneficial to all patients, but for the fortunate ones it does provide significant improvement and sometimes a total cure.

The artificial sphincter is a doughnut-shaped balloon that encircles the urethra. A man who has received an artificial sphincter must operate a pump implanted in his scrotum each time he wants to relieve himself. It is a device that many find satisfactory.

Modified Stamey Procedure

Dr. Thomas Stamey, Professor of Urology at Stanford University School of Medicine, has developed a technique that can cure urinary incontinence caused by prostate removal but not by neurological deterioration or other causes.

This new procedure involves implanting two GoreTex–covered pads of Dacron so that they gently compress the part of the urethra that rests below the pubic arch behind the scrotum, creating a substitute for the sphincter muscle. This allows men to urinate in a normal fashion. Since first developing this technique several years ago, Dr. Stamey has used it on sixty-five patients. The procedure, which takes one to three hours, completely relieved incontinence in fifty-eight of the men—a cure rate of about 90 percent. The men who were not completely cured by the operation have benefited nonetheless, Stamey said, because they are experiencing much less incontinence than before the sphincter surgery.

Penile Clamps

A penile clamp is a clamp that snaps on to the penis and prevents leakage. It is important not to leave it on too long, or it can cause damage to the skin. Patients are advised to take it off every half hour to allow the bladder to empty and to allow the blood flow that is essential for healthy tissue.

Absorbers and Collectors

Many absorbent products and devices are used successfully by patients having problems with urine leakage. The choice depends on the amount of urine leakage and a man's shape, size, and activity level.

There are small drip collectors that fit over the penis and absorb an ounce or more of urine. They feature collectors that can be unobtrusively stored in the pocket.

For men with a problem of uncontrolled and unexpected leakage, there are condom catheters that may be worn with a leg bag during the day and connected to a night bag at bedtime. It is important that this external catheter be fitted and applied correctly.

There are also two-piece pad-and-pant systems that allow a man to have the comfort of a fitted brief and the security of an absorbent pad.

When these products are needed, ask your urologist for a referral to a nurse specialist or a home health supplier with the skills and training to assist you. It is not advisable to select the products on your own.

Skin Care

Since skin care is very important to avoid rashes, use a special cleaner that is available for urinary incontinence. Ask your urologist to recommend one that will allow you to wash many times each day without the drying and irritating effects of most soaps.

There are also moisture-barrier creams and films that may be applied to protect your penis, scrotum, and surrounding skin. Taking this special care will help you to adjust to this problem considerably.

Lifestyle Changes

It is safe to assume that incontinence creates stress for the patient and family, so biofeedback, meditation, and visualization, which are useful to adjust to any form of stress, can be helpful.

Exercise and diet are also important for a male who has a problem with incontinence. If a man eats too much and doesn't get enough exercise, he is likely to gain weight, which will increase pressure on his bladder. Caffeine and alcohol can aggravate incontinence. A proper diet will reduce the problem of constipation without dependence on laxatives. Be aware, too, that drugs usually prescribed for high blood pressure can have a diuretic effect.

As always, it is important to drink a lot of water to help flush out the bladder. To avoid the annoyance of getting up often during the night, cut down on fluids before going to bed (after all, enjoying a good night's sleep was one of the big dividends of having the surgery).

Support Groups

There are many support groups listed in the "Resources" section at the back of this book. If you become incontinent, many men who have experienced this problem will be happy to discuss it with you. They will share their personal experiences and how they are adjusting to incontinence and overcoming its difficulties. They will also share their own sexual problems and other intimate facts that you might not discuss with others. Social interaction is a good way to lift spirits and reduce tension. You will be encouraged by the group to do Kegel exercises and to use other methods to help you.

To not share your feelings with your family and friends is an unwise decision and a surrender to hopelessness and helplessness. Going public with your problem, especially with your loved ones, provides a healing partnership and support that will improve the quality of life after surgery.

Needless to say, your bout with prostate cancer or with other prostate problems has been a challenge to you and your loved ones—but you've made it. You are alive and can now look forward to many more pleasant years. Your brain speaks to your body on a regular basis. Send it positive messages. Maintain an optimistic outlook to have a full and healthful life.

PART V

A Lifestyle for a Healthy Prostate

CHAPTER THIRTEEN

Nutrition

We do well to remember the statement made by Dr. Paul Dudley White, the world-famous heart specialist who cared for former President Dwight Eisenhower after his heart attack: "We were meant to be field animals, to rise with the sun, to be in the open air, to be physically vigorous, and to eat only when hunger dictates."

Growing numbers of health professionals are theorizing that as much as 50 percent of cancer can be prevented or controlled with good nutrition. Roger J. Williams, a foremost nutrition authority, states that well-nourished cells are relatively resistant to outside attacks and that one of the strong hopes for prevention of cancer lies in the field of specialized nutrition.

Patrick Quillin, Vice President of Nutrition for the Cancer Treatment Center of America and author of the book *Treating Cancer with Nutrition*, states, "The cure must come from changing the environment within the body.... The sexually related cancers, such as prostate cancer, seem to be the most responsive to nutrition therapy." He suggests eating fruits and vegetables, especially the most colorful ones. For example, sweet potatoes are better than white potatoes, because their orange color indicates the presence of phytochemicals including beta-carotene. Red grapes are preferable to white grapes, because the red grapes have more cancer-fighting proanthocyanidens. And reach for the reddest tomato, as it is richer in lycopene, another chemical suspected to help prevent prostate cancer.

In addition, fresh vegetables are recommended over cooked, canned, or frozen ones, as these processes can wipe out glutathione—a nutrient that can trigger the body to fight impurities that cause cancer.

Diets rich in animal fat appear to be associated with an increased risk of prostate cancer; there is a strong positive correlation between the consumption of dietary fat and the incidence of prostate cancer worldwide.

DIETARY DEMOGRAPHICS AND PROSTATE CANCER

"The death rate from prostate cancer in the United States is 700 percent higher than that in Hong Kong and 600 percent higher than that in Japan. Populations that eat larger amounts of fat have strikingly higher rates of prostate cancer," according to Curtis Mettlin, Chief of Epidemiology Research at Roswell Park Memorial Institute in Buffalo, New York.

For example, Greek males who eat a low-fat diet have a very low rate of prostate cancer. Not the same for Greek males who emigrate to the United States and develop a taste for our fatty diet. This same peril develops for other immigrants who move to the United States and adopt our high-fat diet.

Alice S. Whitemore, Professor of Epidemiology and Biostatistics at Stanford University School of Medicine, concludes that a statistically significant correlation exists between total fat intake and prostate cancer risk for all ethnic groups. Her research indicates that the incidence of prostate cancer in China and Japan is less than one-tenth as high as that found in African-Americans. The African-American group ate the highest amount of saturated fat. While Asian-Americans have lower rates of prostate cancer than do African-Americans or Caucasians, their rates are higher than those of men living in China or Japan. Professor Whitemore acknowledges that diet is not the only factor in promoting prostate cancer growth, but it does play a key part.

According to Ernest Wynder, President of the American Health Foundation, differences in diet are the only way to explain why some countries have higher rates of prostate cancer than others. It is suspected that fat raises the levels of testosterone and other hormones, which could stimulate the prostate to grow along with any cancer cells that it may harbor. This may explain why African-Americans have a 37 percent higher incidence of prostate cancer than Caucasians do, according to the American Cancer Society. Studies have shown that African-Americans have higher levels of testosterone to begin with; a high-fat diet could further elevate those levels, contributing to a higher rate of prostate cancer.

According to Dr. Stephen Barnes, Associate Professor of Pharmocology and Biochemistry at the University of Alabama, Birmingham, when native-born Japanese men leave their country, where prostate cancer death rates are low, and move to the United States, they become twenty times more susceptible to prostate cancer than if they had stayed in Japan. What could cause such a dramatic increase in risk? The radical change in diet is a prime suspect. Instead of soy-based, low-fat foods, these Japanese emigrants shift to the higher-fat, more meat-based American fare.

FOODS THAT MAY HELP PREVENT PROSTATE CANCER

We are what we eat, it's said. Data continues to bear out the healthful benefits of natural foods and dietary supplements, so it stands to reason that naturally healthy foods make for naturally healthy people.

Soy Products

Is it possible that soy is a magic bean? Soy proteins have been found to inhibit cancer cells from spreading in the body. They are consumed daily by Asian men in their homeland, but rarely in

America. When genistein, a key component of soybeans, was put in a petri dish with prostate cancer cells, it stopped the cancer dead in its tracks. Dr. Stephen Barnes, intrigued by this information, is conducting a study on the effects of soy products involving 80 men with elevated PSA levels.

Dr. Barnes states that recent work done at Johns Hopkins School of Medicine may tie in with his research. There, investigators have identified a gene that controls the creation of a chemical that can help protect men against prostate cancer. If Dr. Barnes can determine a link between soy products and the functioning of that gene, his discovery would be a significant breakthrough.

Two Finnish scientists investigated the possible role of the Japanese diet in prostate health. Japanese men have a lower death rate from prostate cancer than do men from Western cultures, even though in Japan they have about the same incidence of small prostate cancers. The researchers wondered if it were possible that the Japanese diet might keep small prostate cancers from growing into deadly tumors.

The researchers also observed that Seventh-Day Adventist men, who typically eat a lot of lentils, peas, beans, tomatoes, raisins, dates, and dried fruits, have a low death rate from prostate cancer, as do Japanese men living in Hawaii who continue to eat rice and tofu. These foods are rich in isoflavonoids—plant versions of the female sex hormone estrogen—that inhibit the growth of cancer cells in the test tube.

The researchers analyzed blood samples from 14 Japanese men who ate the typical soy-rich Japanese diet and 14 Finnish men who ate the typical dairy-and-meat diet of Finland. The levels of the estrogen-like isoflavonoids were 7 to 114 times higher in the blood of the Japanese men than in the blood of the Finns. The Finnish researchers concluded: "A lifelong high concentration of isoflavo-noids in [blood] plasma… might explain why Japanese men have small latent carcinomas [cancers] that seldom develop to clinical disease."

In another study, 7,999 American men of Japanese ancestry were first examined between 1965 and 1968 and then followed through 1986. During this time period, 174 cases of prostate cancer were recorded in the group, considerably less than the rate in other populations. The researchers observed that rice and tofu were both associated with decreased risk of prostate cancer.

As mentioned earlier, the incidence of clinically diagnosed prostatic cancer ranged from 0.8 cases per 100,000 population in Shanghai, China, to 100.1 per 100,000 among African-Americans in Alameda County, California. It is much more common among Caucasians than Asians (see page34).

Fruits and Vegetables

Many anthropologists believe that our ancestors were mostly vegetarians. Our teeth are designed primarily for plant-based foods, and our intestinal tract is long, which allows for the slow digestion of plant foods that are high in fiber, as opposed to the short digestive tract that is necessary to process meat and to get rid of the resulting toxic wastes hastily. "Populations who eat plant-based diets have a markedly reduced incidence of chronic ills, most notably cancer and heart disease," says Clare Hasler of the University of Illinois.

It is unfortunate that former President Bush expressed a dislike for broccoli. Broccoli and all its vegetable kin—Brussels sprouts, mustard, kale, and collard greens—have an extraordinary power to fight cancer. These cabbage-family vegetables contain potent chemicals called indoles that block harmful carcinogens before they do their dirty work. Brussels sprouts can also help us enhance the natural ability of our bodies to resist cancer-causing agents. This will not only help the prostate but all of the vital body parts.

It appears that vegetables such as these stimulate production of glutathione's transferase, a catalyst that is involved in chemical reactions. Asians tend to eat more broccoli and related types of vegetables than do Americans, which could also contribute to their low rate of prostate cancer.

Fruits and vegetables are delicious as well as nutritious. Their variety is almost limitless. In my case, if anything saves me from putting on weight it is the fact that I use foods from this group as a snack. Many Americans, trying to lose weight to protect their hearts as well as to improve their appearance, are continually on and off fad diets when they could be losing weight by eating sensibly from the basic four food groups (meat and meat alternates; fruits and vegetables; breads and cereals; nonfat dairy products) and cutting down on foods high in fat and low in nutrients. When you feel the urge to eat, try some apples, pears, carrots, celery, or other foods from this group. They will satisfy your appetite and provide your body with premium fuel.

Other studies disclosed that those who ate more folate-rich foods such as fruits and vegetables are less likely to develop colon cancer. Even among animals, those that are deprived of folic acid face a threefold to fourfold increased risk of colon rectal tumors.

Pectins These may help to prevent prostate cancer. Pectin is a coagulating carbohydrate found in the skins of apples, citrus, and other fruits and vegetables. Researchers fed a group of rats with prostate tumors a modified citrus pectin drink, and they fed another group pure water; they observed a 50 percent reduction in the spread of the cancer to the lungs in the pectin group. The experiment made use of a form of the carbohydrate produced in the laboratory, which is not now available to the public. Still, pectin can also lower cholesterol levels considerably—cholesterol, as you will see later, may increase a man's susceptibility to prostate cancer.

Tomatoes A Harvard study of the eating habits of 47,000 men over a period of six years found that those who had at least ten servings of tomato-based foods a week were up to 45 percent less likely to develop prostate cancer. Most of the protection came from eating spaghetti sauce, said Dr. Edward Giovannucci of the Harvard School of Public Health; pizza, which includes layers of tomato sauce, also helped. Tomatoes are the best source of a carotenoid called lycopene, and they are also rich in phytochemicals.

Lycopene may act to block the initiation of the cancerous process. This natural molecule gives tomatoes their red color—the redder the better. Interestingly, earlier studies revealed that prostate cancer is less common in southern Mediterranean countries, such as Italy and Greece, where tomato-based foods are a major part of the diet. Phytochemicals work by disrupting the chemical wedding between two common molecules in cells—a union that can produce a carcinogen. Every slice of tomato and every bite of apricot contains thousands of them. Strawberries, pineapples, and green peppers are also rich in phytochemicals.

Garlic Long recommended as a food to help patients who have coronary artery disease and to avoid a fatal heart attack, garlic is now gaining recognition as a food that will help to ward off prostate cancer. Certain chemicals in garlic, according to recent new studies, show promising results in actually slowing the growth of prostate cancer cells—at least in a test tube.

Vitamins and Minerals

Is it possible that a lack of vitamins poses a risk factor for prostate cancer?

We hear a great deal about vitamins C and E and beta-carotene as antioxidants. Researchers have believed that antioxidants were effective in limiting the early phases of prostate cancer.

However, while recent research does not prove that antioxidant vitamins provide no benefit, it does suggest a need for more study to determine the value of antioxidants. A 1996 study suggested also to put a hold on the use of antioxidants from pills or supplements, indicating that they may be not only a waste of consumers' money but possibly a danger to their health.

It still makes sense to obtain antioxidants naturally from fruits and vegetables. They are especially rich in carotenes. People who eat more of these valuable foods appear to have a lower risk of most cancers.

Wahida Karmally, Director of Nutrition at Columbia University's Irving Center for Clinical Research and spokesperson for the American Dietetic Association, says, "I recommend that men make sure they get a hearty supply of yellow, orange, and dark green fruits and vegetables to get the beta-carotene and vitamin C they need." Sources of monounsaturated fats, like nuts and vegetable oils, can also boost your vitamin E intake.

Vitamin D A lack of vitamin D may lead to the development of prostate cancer. But don't overdo taking vitamin D, as it can be toxic. For men over the age of twenty-five, the recommended dosage is 200 IU (International Units) per day. Get your vitamin D by consuming fortified skim milk, fish, and other foods that are good sources of vitamin D.

Calcium This is another nutrient that may play an important role in prostate health. One theory suggests that calcium may actually diminish the uptake of fatty acids, thus reducing the potential growth of cancer cells in the body. Nonfat milk and leafy green vegetables will help to maintain adequate intakes of calcium (1000 milligrams a day).

Zinc A Chicago urologist, Dr. Irving M. Bush, has observed that men with chronic prostatitis often have low zinc levels in both their prostate fluid and semen and that patients with prostate cancer also have low zinc stores. He reports that patients treated with zinc have shown improvement in their symptoms.

Dr. William R. Fair, a urologist at Sloan-Kettering Memorial Medical Center in New York City, believes that zinc may be important in the prevention of prostatic diseases, but he cautions that the prostate can't pick up and utilize zinc when it is taken by mouth. Even more critical is Dr. E. David Crawford, who asserts from recent laboratory research that adding zinc to prostate cancer cells actually seemed to make them grow faster. As with other treatments, the use of zinc should be discussed with your doctor and should be based on your individual condition.

FAT CONSUMPTION AND PROSTATE CANCER

A study from Harvard University should motivate you to just say no to the enticing-looking cheeseburger or steak. Beginning in 1986, Dr. Edward Giovannucci analyzed diet questionnaires obtained from 47,855 healthy male dentists, pharmacists, and other health professionals. By 1990, prostate cancer had been diagnosed in 300 of them, with 126 advanced cases. Researchers found that the men who ate the most fat had a 79 percent higher risk of developing advanced prostate cancer than those who ate the least fat. Men who consumed the highest quantities of red meat had a 164 percent higher risk of prostate cancer than did those who got most of their protein from fish and poultry without the skin. Fat from dairy products not including saturated fat (which are usually solid fats of animal origin such as meat, whole milk, cream cheese, and butter), monounsaturated fat, and alphalinolenic acid but not linolenic acid were suspected as having a link to advanced cancer risk.

"We need to confirm these results with further studies," cautions Giovannucci. In the meantime, his advice to red meat eaters is: "The less, the better."

Mice injected with human tumors showed slower disease progression when the fat content of their diets was reduced, according to a study performed by Dr. Yu Wang, reported in the *Journal of the National Cancer Institute*. Researchers at Sloan-Kettering Memorial Cancer Center found that human prostate cancer tumors grew only half as fast in laboratory mice getting 2 percent to 20 percent of their calories from fat as in those eating diets with about 50 percent fat—the level eaten by many American men. Additional studies are needed to see how dietary fat may influence progression from latent to invasive prostate cancer, such as in the relationship between dietary fat and sex hormone levels and the fatty acids and/or their metabolites that may promote tumor progression.

Avoiding Animal Fats

Other investigations also indicate that diets heavy in meat may change prostate cancers from dormant to malignant. Since meat poses a threat to the heart and has been associated with cancer, let's look at both meat and meat substitutes. This is an important group, for it is a major source of protein, which our bodies need to replace dead cells and to form new ones. We must have an adequate intake of protein to maintain good health and to recover from illness and injury. But we can do this and still avoid diets high in red meat, which appear to be cancer's preferred fuel.

Saturated fats, such as those found in red meat and whole dairy products, are the elements to avoid. Polyunsaturated fats, such as those found in olive oil, are not considered to put people at a higher risk for cancer.

Poultry and fish are rich in high-quality protein and can be used as inexpensive substitutes for red meat. Legumes, such as dried beans, soybeans, and dried peas, do not contain as high-quality a protein, but when they are eaten with rice, corn, or a little lean meat, their protein can rival that of meat. All grains and dried legumes contain vitamins, fiber, and proteins while having little fat content and no refined sugar (another food that does not contribute to good health). Red meat products, such as lamb, beef, pork, veal, duck, high-fat poultry with skin, dark meat of either chicken or turkey, and organ meats should be avoided.

Whole-milk dairy products, such as butter, milk, cream, cottage cheese, and yogurt, should be cut out, and their low-fat or nonfat counterparts used instead. Egg whites provide a complete protein while all the cholesterol is found in the yolk, so consider using the egg white and discarding the rest.

Seventh-Day Adventists tend not to eat the typical American diet. They generally eat whole grains, vegetables, and nuts and avoid alcohol, tobacco, caffeine-containing beverages, spices, and highly refined foods. Many of them don't eat meat, and their death rate from intestinal cancer is 20 percent below the average in the United States. Studies at the Loma Linda School of Health in California have shown that they also have consistently lower cholesterol levels. A long-term study of 47,000 Seventh-Day Adventists revealed a much lower death rate than for the general population, and those who were strict vegetarians had the lowest death rate.

The studies also showed that Seventh-Day Adventists who reported consuming the most meat, milk, cheese, and eggs were more than three times as likely to die of prostate cancer within twenty years than were Seventh-Day Adventists who said they ate the lowest amounts of those foods. Other studies related to Seventh-Day Adventists revealed that the men who drank two glasses of milk per day had almost twice the risk of developing prostate cancer of those who drank one glass. Three glasses of milk increased the odds even more.

Cholesterol

New studies indicate a strong possibility that foods that impair the heart are also harmful to the prostate. There is reason to suspect a possible association between prostate tumors and cholesterol, because testosterone, which is recognized as promoting tumor growth, has a chemical structure with important similarities to that of cholesterol. There is the possibility that high levels of cholesterol cause excess testosterone production. Animal fats create excess cholesterol in the bloodstream. Foods high in saturated fats include butter, ice cream, cheese, egg yolks, liver, meat, creams, and gravies.

Fat is the main culprit in raising blood cholesterol. It is a dangerous factor in increasing the risk of heart disease.

Body Weight

There are other studies worth keeping in mind when you point your fork toward that juicy steak. A Harvard study of 25,000 men between the ages of forty and seventy-five found that men with waistlines larger than forty-three inches are more than twice as likely to have enlarged prostates that need to be removed as are men with waist measurements of less than thirty-five inches. Higher weights may elevate blood pressure, which can contribute to problems of the enlarged prostate. With animals, hundreds of studies show that if you give them 60 to 80 percent of their normal calorie consumption, they live much longer, with much lower rates of cancer.

The following chart should help you to make the right selection of food.

LOVE-YOUR-HEART FOOD LIST

Food	Portion	Calories	Grams of Saturated Fat	Grams of Soluble Fiber
MEAT GROUP A				
Chicken (white meat, no skin)	3.5 oz.	140	0.4	—
Cod	3.5 oz.	168	0.2	—
Kidney beans	1 cup	230	—	3.0

LOVE-YOUR-HEART FOOD LIST (continued)

Food	Portion	Calories	Grams of Saturated Fat	Grams of Soluble Fiber
Lobster	3.5 oz.	95	0.1	—
Salmon	3.5 oz.	66	2.0	—
Turkey (white meat)	3.5 oz.	175	0.5	—
Tuna (in water)	3.5 oz.	125	1.5	—
MEAT GROUP B				
Beef, round steak	3.5 oz.	259	3.0	—
Ground beef, lean	3.5 oz.	217	7.0	—
Leg of lamb, lean	3.5 oz.	266	3.0	—
Sausage, pork	3.5 oz.	494	3.0	—
MEAT GROUP C				
Bacon	3.5 oz.	578	17.5	—
Frankfurter, beef	2.0 oz.	458	12.9	—
MILK GROUP A				
Cottage Cheese	3.0 oz.	90	0.5	—
Milk, skim	8.0 oz.	44	0.3	—
Yogurt, plain	8.0 oz.	113	0.2	—
MILK GROUP B				
Cheese, whole-milk	1.0 oz.	115	5.0	—
Milk, whole (3.5 percent fat)	8.0 oz.	80	5.0	—
Yogurt, fruit	8.0 oz.	150	5.0	—
MILK GROUP C				
Ice cream	1 cup	165	14.5	—
Mayonnaise	1 Tbsp.	101	1.5	—
Pie, chocolate cream	⅛ pie	265	17.0	—

LOVE-YOUR-HEART FOOD LIST (continued)

Food	Portion	Calories	Grams of Saturated Fat	Grams of Soluble Fiber
VEGETABLE GROUP A				
Broccoli	½ cup	27	—	1.0
Corn, cooked	½ cup	192	—	1.5
Peas	½ cup	58	—	2.0
Potato, baked, medium	1 potato	92	—	2.0
VEGETABLE GROUP B				
Carrots, raw	½ cup	96	—	0.5
Lettuce	½ cup	13	—	0.2
Tomato, raw	1 medium	92	—	0.2
VEGETABLE GROUP C				
Avocado	1 medium	369	5.0	—
GRAIN GROUP A				
Bread, whole wheat	1 slice	76	—	3.0
Cornmeal	1 cup	433	—	4.0
Oat bran, dry	1 cup	255	—	6.0
Oatmeal, cooked	1 cup	132	—	2.0
40 percent bran flakes	1 cup	106	—	1.0
Flour, all-purpose	1 cup	419	—	2.0
Tortillas, corn	1 tortilla	65	—	1.0
GRAIN GROUP B				
Spaghetti, cooked	1 cup	182	0.5	—
Bread, white	1 slice	76	0.3	—
GRAIN GROUP C				
Angel food cake	⅛ cake	161	0.2	—

BREADS AND CEREALS

If yours is a typical American family, each of you will have a slice of toast for breakfast, two slices of bread in a sandwich for lunch, and perhaps another slice of bread or a roll for dinner. Because bread is so common in our diet and can provide good fuel for our bodies, we need guidance in making a wise choice (as if we don't have enough decisions to make in the course of a day!). I recently counted over fifty brands of bread in our favorite supermarket.

First, reject all brands from which the most nutritious parts of the wheat kernel have been removed. The kernel is made up of three parts. The first is the outer covering, or bran, a rough, many-layered shield rich in crude fiber. Next comes the starchy mass called the endosperm, and then, deep inside, the tiny embryo, or wheat germ, which Mother Nature has wisely provided with all the nutrients needed to spark its growth into a new wheat plant.

White bread is made from the endosperm, the least nutritious part of the kernel, with the bran and the wheat germ thrown away. White flour was being produced in Greece at least as early as 500 B.C.; by A.D. 50 , its production was widespread. Fortunately for the poor, it was a wealthy people's bread, but by the seventeenth century, practically everyone was eating it. Bakers now try to tempt us to eat bread made from this flour by claiming it is "enriched." While it is true that several vitamins and minerals are added to it, they do not nearly make up for all the good that was taken out.

Since it contains the nutrition of all parts of the kernel, whole wheat flour can be thought of as nutritional gold. Removal of the bran and germ in order to appeal to the American palate and to increase the shelf life of the bread is inexcusable. Unaware that for economic reasons we are being deprived of valuable nutrients, many of us raise our families on white bread.

When we eat white flour, we are depriving ourselves of the wheat bran, which provides many valuable nutrients as well as fiber. If we ate the typical meal of the African villager, including cornmeal, beans, bananas, and potatoes, or if we ate a lot of fruit, vegetables, and grains high in fiber, we would be protecting our bodies against a lot of health problems. Since most of us don't eat a well-balanced diet, eating bread with the bran intact will help us avoid the many problems that a diet low in fiber can cause. These problems include constipation, cancer of the colon and rectum (of which the United States has almost the highest rate in the world), appendicitis, hemorrhoids, varicose veins, diverticulosis, and coronary heart disease. By forcing the liver to convert cholesterol into bile salts and subsequently excrete them, a high-fiber diet reduces the amount of cholesterol in the bloodstream.

Cereals have long been very important in the diets of people throughout the world. If we take the time to read labels and make a proper selection, cereals can play an important role in our diets as well. In many parts of the world today, cereals supply 80 percent or more of the total caloric intake as well as valuable amounts of nutrients. This group includes cornmeal, grits, rice, macaroni, and spaghetti.

It's wise to serve cereal made from whole grains, such as rolled oats and whole wheat. It isn't difficult to mix up a batch of good natural foods such as wheat germ, bran, rolled oats, nuts, and raisins to provide your family with a nutritious breakfast. If you don't have time to prepare this, look for the granola type of cereal, preferably one without sugar or coconut. Coconut is very rich in saturated fat, and people who use it as a main staple in their diets have as many coronary heart problems as Americans do.

It is ironic that poor, rural people often have a much more nutritious diet than those of us who live in this wealthy modern society. We Americans seem to be consistent in doing things wrong. Despite strong evidence that fiber plays an important part in reducing cholesterol levels and protecting against atherosclerosis, our consumption of fiber-rich foods has been decreasing for the past sixty years. For the sake of our nation's health, let's hope that with the new information available this trend will be reversed.

NUTRITION AND GENERAL HEALTH

The 1988 Surgeon General's Report on Nutrition and Health, which draws on 2,000 studies, states, "Diet helped account for more than two-thirds of the 2.1 million deaths in the U.S. last year. Poor nutritional habits are strongly implicated in five of the nation's top ten killers: coronary heart disease, stroke, atherosclerosis, diabetes, and some cancers." Poor nutritional habits are also highly suspect in contributing to prostate cancer. While awaiting the results of medical researchers, it makes sense to be more selective in our food. Yes, the fork may very well be deadlier than the sword!

In a survey of more than 3,400 physicians, many agreed that "diet has an important role in disease prevention, and in many cases medication could be reduced or eliminated if patients followed a recommended diet"; they also agreed that doctors should spend more time exploring dietary habits during physicals. However, many physicians fall short in doing so. Survey coordinator Barbara Levins, Director of the Nutrition Information Center in New York Hospital–Cornell Medical Center in New York, responded to the survey results by suggesting that perhaps competence in nutrition should be demonstrated before licensure to practice medicine is granted. Maybe that is an idea whose time has come.

As Dr. Michael Thun of the American Cancer Society says, "There is more and more evidence that grandmother was right: eating a diet high in fresh fruits and vegetables and low in fat is a good thing for a variety of illnesses, and now it may be beneficial for cancer too."

CHAPTER FOURTEEN

Exercise and Relaxation

It doesn't make sense to concern yourself with preventing prostate problems while neglecting the rest of the body. Chapter 13 covered diet and nutrition as factors in developing a healthy body and mind. This chapter will cover two other aspects of a well-balanced lifestyle that may contribute to overall good health: exercise and stress management.

EXERCISE

Modern man appears to be a lazy animal, inclined to put out the minimum energy necessary for survival. It is a sign of our affluence that special exercise programs are needed to compensate for our daily inactivity. No longer do we have to cut wood to cook food or to provide warmth for our family. All we have to do is strike a match or push a button. It's rare to see someone washing or polishing a car when it's so easy just to drive through a car wash. When I see the garbage collectors getting out of their trucks to collect refuse, I think how fortunate they are to have a job that requires so much physical activity. They will probably outlive lawyers, ministers, teachers, and others who work in sedentary occupations.

In addition to being good for our general health, there are some studies that suggest a relationship between exercise and prostate cancer. A study by I. M. Lee showed that men who burned 4,000 calories per week or more (the equivalent of an hour's active workout) had a much lower incidence of prostate cancer than did men who burned fewer than 1,000 calories per week. Investigators theorized that increased physical activity produced lower levels of prostate-stimulating androgens.

Researchers in Dallas assessed the physical fitness of 13,344 initially healthy men and women, and then followed them for an average of eight years. They found that even mild exercise postpones death and that regular exercise may help to prevent cancer.

The Dallas study was not the first to suggest that exercise will ward off cancer. There have also been studies done on Iowa farmers and Harvard alumni, both of which found that the death rate from cancer was highest in those who exercised the least.

The reasons for this are not clear. Perhaps by speeding food (with its potential carcinogens) through the intestine, exercise may curb the risk of colon and rectal cancer. Exercise may also augment diverse immune defenses.

Exercise improves circulation, raises blood levels, and improves oxygen utilization. The prostate gland benefits from both the increased blood flow and the improved quality of blood that reaches it. More studies are needed to establish a stronger connection between exercise and prostate health, but a strong suspicion exists among many medical investigators that the connection is indeed there.

Just one precaution: You should not ride a bicycle if you are scheduled for a PSA test that day, as it could affect your test result. The same caution applies to water skiing and horseback riding prior to having your PSA evaluated. Similarly, some urologists advise against having sexual relations prior to taking a PSA test (although there is no evidence that it changes results significantly).

Among men over age fifty-five, researchers find that many of the physical symptoms of aging are merely the result of inactivity.

Their findings also indicate that even moderate exercise can retard the effects of aging and even reverse them. The important thing at this age is to keep moving.

One group of Americans who seek out opportunities to exercise are doctors, especially heart specialists. They avoid elevators and run up and down stairs as they make their daily rounds in the hospitals. Dr. Edward Bortz, past president of the American Medical Association, states, "I take vigorous exception to the prophets of doom who see only the degeneration of the human body with the passing of time. It begins to appear that exercise is the master conditioner for the healthy and the major therapy of the ill."

THE NEED TO REDUCE STRESS

Is it possible that the same components (anger, stress, and insecurity) that have been proven to be a contributing factor to coronary artery disease could be setting up males for prostate cancer? Experts agree that overreacting to daily stress, when combined with poor eating habits and lack of exercise, can deal the final blow to the body's autoimmune and other life-preserving systems. As a result, stress can well be considered the number one public health threat of the 1990s.

According to one survey, during any six-month period, approximately 29 million Americans, or 18 percent of the population, will have a stress-related alcohol, drug abuse, or mental health disorder. Over 57 million Americans suffer from stress-related hypertension. Over the last several years, over $13 billion has been spent per year on medical care for stress-related stroke victims. And more than one in four Americans suffer from some form of stress-related cardiovascular disease. Men appear to be particularly susceptible to the effects of stress, which possibly may explain the relatively lower life expectancy of males.

Stress Is Inevitable

In a now-famous study, University of Washington psychiatrist Thomas Holmes determined that the single, common denominator for all types of stress is change in an individual's life pattern. This means that any change in your regular pattern of living—including taking a vacation, divorce, getting a raise, the death of a spouse, buying a house, and even Christmas—creates stress, which may be positive or negative. Any out-of-the-ordinary event creates stress.

In an attempt to measure the impact of life-changing events, Holmes and psychologist Richard Rahe asked 5,000 people to rate the amount of social readjustment required for various events. The result is the widely used Holmes-Rahe scale. Here is a sample of what they found:

Life Event	Stress Points
Death of spouse	100
Divorce	73
Marital separation	65
Imprisonment	63
Marriage	50
Pregnancy	40
Buying a house	31
Christmas	12

Holmes showed that in a sample of 88 young doctors, those who had a total life-stress rating of 300 or more units had a 70 percent chance of suffering ulcers, psychiatric disturbances, cancer, heart attacks, broken bones, and similar difficulties within a year. Those who scored under 200 had only a 37 percent incidence of health problems within a year. Over the years, this scale has proved to be a good predictor of individuals who would suffer future stress. The scale has proved so reliable that by tallying up the life stress points of healthy football players, Holmes and Rahe were able to predict which ones would be injured during the next season.

If a person can understand what is causing him to feel depressed or upset and can learn to manage it effectively, then stress may no longer be feared. Stress management is essential because stress is unavoidable. "We live in a world of uncertainties," says Dr. Herbert Benson of Harvard Medical School, "everything from the nuclear threat, to corporation takeovers, to job insecurity, to worry over the economy and everything else."

Past studies have identified the type A personality, which is described by Dr. Meyer Friedman as a person with an intense drive to succeed while battling against the clock. In doing so, this person is setting himself up for a fatal heart attack.

Dr. Friedman feels that the type A factor is more important than exercise, diet, or heredity, although he cautions against a diet rich in animal fat and cholesterol, especially for type A men and women.

The type B man does not have the traits of the type A. He is less likely to suffer an impatient sense of time or need to boast about achievements. He will play for fun and relaxation, not a will to dominate, and he will relax without guilt and work without undue drive.

How stress affects each individual depends on whether he is type A or type B. The most dramatic proof of the influence of stress on coronary heart disease was provided by doctors Friedman and Rosenman, who used behavior patterns to predict which subjects in a group of 3,500 would develop heart disease.

After over eight years of follow-up, they found that type A subjects had more than twice as much heart disease as type B subjects, who go through life at a more sensible and relaxed pace. Type A subjects had twice as much anginal pain, twice as many heart attacks, five times as many recurring heart attacks, and twice as many fatal heart events. Among subjects who died of causes other than heart disease, the coronary arteries of the type A subject almost always showed far more disease than those of the type B subject. Among the subjects considered the most relaxed but whose cholesterol level was 225, not one had a heart attack.

Type A people have much higher cholesterol levels than type B people. Dr. Friedman showed that tax accountants' blood cholesterol levels rose with the stress of tax deadlines and fell when the deadlines had passed. Since the accountants were eating the same types of food during both periods and did not alter smoking or exercising habits, he felt the change in cholesterol levels could be due only to the added emotional stress.

Doctors Friedman and Rosenman also found that individuals with extreme type A behavior patterns exhibited every blood fat and hormonal abnormality associated with heart disease, abnormalities that many cardiologists believe precede and possibly cause coronary heart disease. The researchers concluded that the type A behavior pattern itself gave rise to the abnormalities.

Later studies of the type A and type B personalities have implicated the person with a high hostility factor. Everyone is burdened with some form of hidden anger and resentment that in turn expresses itself negatively in their life. Hidden anger tends to seep into our daily experience without our knowledge.

Once the anger is lodged in the subconscious, it seems to take over. Studies by Redford B. Williams, Jr., of the Duke University Medical Center in Durham, North Carolina, suggest that high scores on a psychological test designed to measure hostility are associated with high risk of heart disease from all causes. These studies show that it is not the hard-driving workaholic who is at risk but the hard-driving workaholic who is also angry, hostile, and distrustful.

His research also found that a study group of doctors with high scores on a hostility test given during medical school were more likely to die during the twenty-five-year follow-up period than were their more relaxed peers. Only 2 percent of physicians with low or average hostility scores died, while 14 percent of physicians with above average hostility died during the same period.

In a related study, researchers followed a group of 118 lawyers who were given the Minnesota Multiphasic Personality Inventory test. Twenty years later, those with the higher hostility scores died at a rate 412 times higher than those with low scores.

Managing Stress

During the last days of World War II, President Truman was asked how he managed to bear up so calmly under the stresses of the presidency. "I have a foxhole in my mind," he replied, explaining that just as a soldier retreats into his foxhole for protection and respite, he periodically retreated into his mental "foxhole," where he allowed nothing to bother him. In doing so he was following the wisdom of Marcus Aurelius, who wrote, "Nowhere, either with more quiet or more freedom from trouble, does a man retire more than into his own soul."

Learn to Relax One technique that has helped many handle stress is meditation. Studies indicate that if practiced regularly, relaxation exercises can produce a significant lowering of blood pressure and can improve a person's sense of well-being and his ability to cope with his world.

Prayer is a form of meditation, and some people believe that regular churchgoers have fewer heart attacks than those who do not regularly attend their church. An Israeli study showed that among people who went to synagogues, 24 per 1,000 suffered heart attacks as compared to 56 per 1,000 for people who rarely went. Well-documented studies of Y. Kemi evaluating instances of spontaneous cancer remission suggest that a strong faith, religious or otherwise, was the common determining factor among the patients.

Dr. Benson of Harvard is a firm believer in exercise and meditation to help a person to relax. He believes that it can help a type A individual to avoid heart attacks. Could it possibly help to avoid prostate cancer? Many believe that it can. According to Dr. Louis

E. Kapolow, "The best strategy for avoiding stress is to learn how to relax." Unfortunately, many people try to relax at the same pace that they lead the rest of their lives. For a while, tune out your worries about time, productivity, and doing right. You will find satisfaction in just being, without striving. Find activities that give you pleasure and that are good for your mental and physical well-being. Forget about always winning. Focus on relaxation, enjoyment, and health. Be good to yourself.

Get Active Dr. Kapolow also suggests trying physical activity. Along with many other medical professionals, he recommends that when you are nervous, angry, or upset that you try releasing the pressure through physical activity. Physical exercise will relieve that uptight feeling. Relax and turn the frowns into smiles. Remember that your body and your mind work together.

When you do engage in a competitive game, remember that it is all right to lose. As Dr. Friedman advises, avoid playing with a type A person. If you do, modify your behavior and try to act as a type B personality (if you're not one already). After all, who will remember a year from now whether you won or lost the match?

The next time you wake up in a bad mood and want to change it, think about taking an aerobics class or going for a run; it could really make a difference. Exercise was rated by the general population and by psychotherapists as the best strategy to change a bad mood. Television watching, on the other hand, was found to be unsuccessful in lifting one's mood.

Schedule time for both work and recreation. Play can be just as important to your well-being as work; you need a break from your daily routine to just relax and have fun.

One way to keep from getting bored, sad, and lonely is to go where it's all happening. Sitting alone can make you feel frustrated. Instead of feeling sorry for yourself, get involved and become a participant. Offer your services in neighborhood or volunteer organizations. Help yourself by helping other people. Get involved in the world and with the people around you, and you'll find they will be attracted to you. You're on your way to making new friends and enjoying new activities.

Make a Schedule Trying to take care of everything at once can seem overwhelming, and, as a result, you may not accomplish anything. Instead, make a list of what tasks you have to do, then do one at a time, checking them off as they're completed. Give priority to the most important ones and do those first.

- Leave enough time between activities so that you minimize overlap.
- Schedule only as many tasks each day as you can reasonably finish without pressure.
- Leave time in your schedule for the unexpected.
- Leave early enough so that you need not rush to get where you are going, even if this means rising 20 minutes earlier in the morning.
- If you are usually too busy, leave details to someone else whenever possible (the income tax return, fixing your car, office details).

Other Ways to Reduce Stress Do other people upset you, particularly when they don't do things your way? Try cooperation instead of confrontation; it's better than fighting and always being "right." A little give and take on both sides will reduce the strain and make you both feel more comfortable.

A good cry can be a healthy way to bring relief to your anxiety, and it might even prevent a headache or other physical consequence. Take some deep breaths; that activity also releases tension.

You can't always run away, but you can "dream the impossible dream." A quiet country scene painted mentally, or on canvas, can take you out of the turmoil of a stressful situation. Change the scene by reading a good book or playing beautiful music to create a sense of peace and tranquility. Of considerable help to me is that each day I will take at least 20 minutes to create a scene in my mind of the ocean, which is my favorite spot to relax and to regenerate my enthusiasm for whatever project I am involved in.

It helps to talk to someone about your concerns and worries. Perhaps a friend, family member, teacher, or counselor can help you see your problem in a different light. If you feel your problem is serious, you might seek professional help from a psychologist, psychiatrist, or social worker. Knowing when to ask for help may avoid more serious problems later. No man is an island and can stand alone.

If a problem is beyond your control and cannot be changed at the moment, don't fight the situation. Learn to accept things as they are—for now—until such time as you can change them. As expressed at Alcoholics Anonymous meetings, "God grant me the serenity to accept the things that I cannot change, the courage to change the things I can, and the wisdom to know the difference."

Take care of yourself. Get enough rest and eat well. If you are irritable and tense from lack of sleep or if you are not eating correctly, you have less ability to deal with stressful situations. If stress repeatedly keeps you from sleeping, you should ask your doctor to help.

Stress and Sex

There is do doubt about it: stress will put a hold on your sex life. Most men realize that their stomachs can become upset when they are under stress; but, assays Dr. Richard E. Berger, a urology professor at University of Washington Medical School in Seattle, "they don't realize that erections can be affected by the same thing."

In our society, the male is indoctrinated to achieve at everything, and sex is no exception. Many boys and men are brainwashed with many false myths into believing that they should always be ready to have sex and that all intimate contact should result in sexual relations. During adolescence, when the penis often knows only one position (rigid) and ejaculations are very strong, all seems well. But moving past the adolescent age and becoming older, men discover that it takes longer to achieve an erection and it is not as full or hard. As we age, the hormones no longer gallop through our bodies at the same pace as when we were younger; we should not feel embarrassed by the fact that we are no longer sex machines.

However, performance anxiety (fear of not being able to perform sexually) is certainly not a new event and has been referred to since ancient times. This fear concerns not only the middle-aged man but, as doctors now realize, the eighty- to ninety-year-old male as well. Problems in performing, as sexual investigators Masters and Johnson and Dr. Ruth are quick to point out, are often due to the emotions of the individual.

Erectile dysfunction is certainly not a unique problem. (By the way, erectile dysfunction is a more acceptable term than impotence. The term impotence creates a mental picture of a male being sterile or weak with little vigor or power. In 1992, the National Institutes of Health defined erectile dysfunction as the inability to sustain or achieve an erection.) According to the American Foundation for Urologic Disease, it affects ten million to thirty million men in the United States ages forty to seventy. You should discuss this problem openly with your mate and doctor, as disclosing your difficulty will be very helpful in overcoming this most annoying disturbance. Stress. Contrary to prevailing feeling, however, it is not always a condition related to emotional disorders or stress. Seventy percent of the cases of erectile dysfunction are physical and due to a medical problem, such as blockage in the arteries that furnish blood to the penis. A low HDL level is also associated with the problem. Diabetes, neurological disorders, diseases of the erectile tissue of the penis, as well as pelvic surgery can also be blamed for this condition. Also, for many males, this problem could have existed before any type of treatment began.

Kidney and liver problems, hormonal abnormalities, and the side effects caused by prescription drugs taken for cholesterol, high blood pressure, or other illnesses frequently create or compound this problem. Excessive use of alcohol, heavy smoking, and drug abuse are also on the list of culprits. Fortunately, most cases of erectile dystenction are curable or controllable. There are many ways for a man to overcome this distress.

Tests will be given to determine if the arterial blood flow is adequate for an erection. Your doctor will want to make sure that the blood vessels in your penis are still capable of responding. The nerves in the area of your penis will be evaluated to establish if they have satisfactory sensation.

A WELL-BALANCED LIFE

It is difficult to point out the main factor that will contribute to a healthy heart and perhaps a healthy prostate as well. Exercise? Diet? The control of stress? A good example is the study of coronary heart disease among Seventh-Day Adventists who have an extremely low rate of heart disease (see Chapter 13). Nutritionists are quick to say the cause was diet, but other investigators think that perhaps the men were protected by their close-knit, family-oriented social structure, which provided a lot of tender loving care.

According to a study of 3,809 Japanese men aged thirty to seventy-four years old, those who maintained the traditional lifestyle of close family and social contacts have a reduced risk of coronary heart disease. In fact, the investigators found that Japanese-American men with the greatest social isolation and most traumatic life events had twice the risk of dying of coronary heart disease. It seems that people need people. Perhaps this factor is as important as the level of fat in your diet. Socrates said it so well: "There is no illness of the body apart from the mind."

PART VI

On the Horizon

CHAPTER FIFTEEN

New and Evolving Therapies

The man suffering from the effects of an enlarged prostate or prostate cancer can take some comfort in the fact that help is on the way. Medical researchers are working at universities and hospitals to improve screening tests to identify problems at their earliest stages and to then destroy the cancer or otherwise treat the condition.

Additional investigation is needed to determine why some prostate cancers grow slowly and why some are aggressive and spread rapidly to other organs in the body, especially to the bones. It is still unknown why prostate cancer incidence rates are 37 percent higher for African-American males than Caucasian males. The effects of diet, exercise, stress, and environment have to be further explored. When, how, and whether the patient should be treated require more definite guidelines. With the graying of America, these answers have never been so needed.

There are still a lot of unlocked mysteries pertaining to the cause of prostate problems and the most effective way to treat the individual patient, but progress is being made. It is in fact very possible that by the time you have read this book, a new drug or other form of treatment will have been discovered.

Research is now underway to see what stimulates the growth of new blood vessels that furnish tiny cancers with nutrients so they can grow larger and eventually destroy their hosts. If this growth can be discouraged and the blood vessels can somehow be prevented from spreading elsewhere to the body, then the battle against prostate cancer will take a giant step forward.

Needless to say, we all look forward to the day when a magic bullet will be developed that will eliminate problems associated with BPH and prostate cancer. In the meantime, there are many products and programs being developed.

PROSTASURE

A new blood test called ProstAsure is looking very promising. Recent clinical tests indicate a 90 percent accuracy rate in detecting prostate cancer. According to Dr. Oesterling, "ProstAsure represents a significant advancement in both sensitivity and specificity of tumor detection." It is not yet approved by the FDA, but it is available to physicians nationwide for investigational use.

According to researchers speaking at an American Urological Association annual meeting, preliminary research shows that ProstAsure vastly reduces the number of false positive results when compared with currently used methods. They believe that ProstAsure could decrease the need for costly and invasive biopsies by as much as 75 percent.

NEW DRUGS

There is a lot of hope on the horizon for new chemical solutions. The following sections describe a few new drugs.

Suramin

Suramin is a bright spot for men whose cancer has spread beyond the prostate, especially if they haven't done well with hormone therapy, according to Dr. Charles Myers, head of the Cancer Center at the University of Virginia. It works by blocking the activity of a growth factor that tumors need in order to grow new blood vessels—it literally chokes the tumor.

Suramin works in 30 to 50 percent of men who take it, but the side effects are significant and include swelling of the ankles and kidney changes. It can even be fatal. It appears that a newer way of using this drug with smaller doses for a shorter period of time has resulted in better results and fewer side effects.

Ketaconozole

Ketaconozole is a drug that has been used to treat fungal infections. As with Suramin, it is used by urologists when prostate cancer has not responded to standard hormone therapy. Some patients have good results when using Ketaconozole, but it does create major side effects such as serious liver damage. Therefore, the person taking it must have regular blood tests to check liver function.

Strontium and Adriamycin

The standard androgen-blocking drugs cannot control cancer at this stage. Researchers have been seeking new drugs to stop the progression of the cancer and relieve the pain. It appears that a group at the M. D. Anderson Cancer Center in Houston may have done just that. In recent trials, strontium 89, a pain-relieving drug, and adriamycin, an antibiotic with antitumor activity, showed good results in relieving pain and reducing the spread of cancer as evidenced by PSA levels.

GENE THERAPY

According to an October 5, 1994, article in *Time* magazine, researchers have found a faulty gene that may be a cause of most prostate cancer. The defect prevents cells from making an enzyme that fights off carcinogenic chemicals. The discovery could lead to better blood tests and even a drug treatment for the disease.

Gene therapy is a new and provocative means of treating malignancy. Although gene therapy is in its infancy, it offers the potential of transferring healthy genes into cancer cells to replace faulty genes.

At this time, the ideal gene for this has not been clearly identified. Many genes are capable of altering the biological behavior of prostate cancer. Researchers are persevering to select the appropriate gene to do the job.

It is exciting to think of a gene that could treat local cancer and prevent it from spreading. The ultimate success of a prostate cancer gene therapy will depend on a thorough investigation of the biology of the tumor and careful planning of an effective intervention.

"One of the attractive aspects of gene therapy for prostate cancer is that the gland lies just inside the rectum and is easy to biopsy. This would also facilitate the delivery of gene therapy. While gene therapy will still be a complicated procedure, we believe that this is the type of research that will lead to a cure of this disease," says Dr. Ralph W. deVere White, Medical Director of the Mathews Foundation and an active proponent of gene therapy.

"Our aim will be to identify the genetic abnormality that predisposes patients to prostate cancer, screen for that abnormality, and then correct it by directly replacing genes in the prostate. Through this kind of therapy, we feel that the problem of prostate cancer will be defeated."

In an exciting breakthrough, researchers at the National Institutes of Health and Johns Hopkins University have identified a gene called KA11 that prevents cancer cells from metastasizing. So far, it has only been shown to do so in laboratory animals injected with human prostate cancer, but it does offer encouragement.

IMMUNITY BOOSTERS (BIOLOGICAL THERAPY)

Immunity boosters (also called biological therapy) have great potential in the medical treatment of cancer patients. Immune cells that are armed with a toxin may be able to latch onto prostate cancer cells and kill them. A better method may be to vaccinate the body with genes that stimulate production of immune cells that will fight the cancer.

GUIDED ANTIBODIES

This is a process by which synthetic disease-fighting antibodies will attach to prostate cancer cells and destroy them with a toxin. This is a new area of research, but with not much hope at the present time, according to Dr. Peter Scardeno, Chairman of the Urology Department at Baylor College of Medicine in Houston. It hasn't worked on animals yet, but one antibody, CYT 356, is already being developed.

IMMUNOTHERAPY

Immunotherapy is another treatment wherein an attempt is made to build up the patient's immune system against cancer. It appears to have great potential for the future.

Most encouraging is the development of the first vaccine for prostate cancer, which began testing in May 1995. This will be an entirely new approach to treating this problem. The new treatment will be given to men following prostatectomy, to prompt their immune systems to hunt down cancer cells throughout their bodies. "We are trying to prevent the cancer from coming back," said Dr. Jonathan Simons of Johns Hopkins Medical School.

The treatment is called a vaccine because it manipulates the body's own natural disease-fighters to combat an illness. Most vaccines are given to prevent disease, but this one is intended for use after a disease is already established. The vaccine is actually custom-made using the cancer patient's own cells. The doctors save the cancer tissue that is removed during the surgery, and they then insert a copy of a gene into these cancer cells. This gene makes a protein that activates disease-fighting white blood cells that will attack the cancerous cells.

THE NEED FOR MORE RESEARCH

Prostate cancer research has been underfunded in the past, but there is currently a feeling of optimism, because many knowledgeable legislators are working diligently to remedy that lack of funding. They are submitting bills to provide funds to find out what causes this disease and how it can be cured.

According to Mary Lou Wright, Executive Director of the Mathews Foundation, Congress only appropriated $39 million for prostate cancer research in fiscal year 1993. In comparison, $400 million was appropriated for breast cancer research. Breast cancer kills about 46,000 women each year, as opposed to about 40,400 male prostate cancer deaths.

For an even more startling contrast, it is interesting to note that AIDS, which kills about 18,000 persons each year, received research funding of $1.2 billion for fiscal year 1993.

In fact, prostate cancer receives less than 1 percent of research funds allocated by the National Institutes of Health. Why does this disease, which is second only to lung cancer in the number of male deaths annually, merit so little research funding?

The reality is that it takes research to find the most important answers. And meaningful research requires adequate funding.

It makes economic sense to spend more research money on a disease that entails such high treatment costs. A recently published study covering a seventy-five-year period reported that every dollar invested in medical research saved $13 in health care costs, absenteeism, and lost productivity. Prostate cancer is at epidemic levels. Most of us know at least one victim of this awesome disease. If any man lives long enough, he will probably be a victim, too.

A study by researchers at the Johns Hopkins Medical Institution provides more motivation for the U.S. government and other funding sources to loosen up their purse strings. It predicts that by the year 2000, the annual increase in deaths from prostate cancer will be 37 percent, while new cases will soar by 90 percent per year.

CONCLUSION

If this book helps you to understand the problems you may be experiencing from an enlarged or cancerous prostate gland and assists you in making the right choices to defeat this problem, then the time spent in its preparation was well worth it.

Your chances of living a full and healthful life are better than ever and improving all the time. Despite complications that do occur, a UCLA study provides evidence that prostate cancer patients can enjoy a general sense of health and well-being similar to that of a man who has not experienced this problem. The major activities in the patients' daily lives are not compromised after prostate cancer therapy, regardless of which treatment they have chosen.

The number of centenarians in the United States has doubled every decade since 1970. You have an excellent chance of joining this select group and becoming a centenarian in the 21st century if you engage in a healthy regimen of exercise, diet, and relaxation.

If you haven't been living a healthy lifestyle, don't expect your physician to patch up the damage you have done to yourself by improper diet, neglecting to exercise, excessive use of alcohol, smoking, and too much stressful living. But if you now employ the health recommendations provided in this book and develop sound health practices, your probability of living a healthy and satisfying life will be increased considerably.

If you are in your sixties or seventies, your generation has been through a lot. You have paid your dues many times, including living through the Depression years and World War II. You have most likely raised a family and are now helping to raise your grandchildren. You have much more to contribute, and you are certainly entitled to enjoy your golden years. Go for it.

Glossary

abdomen The lower part of the body that contains the liver, stomach, intestines, and spleen.

acidphosphate Enzyme made in the prostate gland.

acute Signifying sharpness or severity.

acute urinary retention Condition where person is suddenly unable to void his urine.

adenoma A benign tumor in which the cells form recognizable glandular structure.

adenocarcinoma A cancer that develops in the glandular lining of an organ. More than five percent of prostate cancers are this type.

adjuvent therapy Treatment that is given to supplement the main therapy.

adrenal gland These are the glands located above the kidney that produce several kinds of hormones including sex hormones.

age specific references Normal values of laboratory studies that consider variations as they occur with advancing age.

alkaline phosphatase Enzyme that is produced in the liver and bones. It helps the urologist to determine if a prostate cancer has spread to the bones.

American Board of Urology A board that has its objective to assist the public by making sure of the competency of the specialist in urology. It issues certificates to the accepted candidates and holds the power to revoke their certificate. They prepare lists of the doctors that are certified as urologists.

androgens Hormones secreted by the testes and adrenals that cause the male traits as a deep voice, hair on the body, and the production of sperm.

anesthesia Using a substance or medication to prevent pain during surgery or other painful form of treatment.

anterior Part of an organ structure.

antibiotic A medication to destroy germs that can cause infection.

atherosclerosis Commonly called hardening of the arteries, it causes the artery walls to become thick and irregular from deposits (called plaque or cholesterol) and other substances. It is a major health problem.

artery A blood vessel that carries oxygenated blood from the heart to bodily tissues.

bacteria Single-celled microscopic organisms that can cause infection or inflammation.

bacterial prostatitis Infection in the prostate gland that is caused by bacteria.

balloon dilation A technique that is used for treatment of BPH. A catheter with a balloon at one end is inserted through the urethra and then inflated to open up the obstruction.

benign A growth that is not cancerous.

benign prostatic hyperplasia Nonmalignant excessive growth of prostate cells.

beta carotene A nutrient found in foods such as vegetables and fruit that is considered important for good health.

biopsy Sample of tissue that is removed to be examined under a microscope to see if it contains cancerous cells.

bladder The organ where the urine is stored before it is eliminated from the body.

bladder spasms Painful squeezing of the bladder in response to irritation or injury, usually occurs following surgery of the prostate.

blood clot When the blood thickens to form a solid mass inside a blood vessel.

blood count Measure of the number of red cells in the body that carry oxygen to the tissues.

bone marrow The spongy inside of the bones of the body that produces blood.

bone scan By injecting a radioactive chemical it highlights any bone changes that may indicate cancer.

BPH (Benign Prostatic Hyperplasia) The noncancerous enlargement of the prostate.

brachytherapy The form of radiation therapy in which radioactive pellets are inserted into the prostate.

cancer The uncontrolled growth of cells that if left untreated can spread and eventually destroy the body.

capsule Structure in which something is enclosed, such as the prostate.

cardiovascular Referring to the heart, the blood vessels, coronary arteries and circulatory functions.

catheter A hollow tube used to inject or withdraw fluids from the body.

CAT Scan The use of x-rays and computer technology to do an imaging of the body to provide a cross-section picture to help the doctor make his diagnosis.

chemotherapy Treatment of cancer using chemicals to deter the growth of the malignant cells.

cholesterol A soft, fat-like substance found in all your body's cells. It is used to form cell membranes, some hormones, and other needed tissue.

chronic bacterial prostatitis The bacterial infection of the prostate that persists over a long period.

Computed Tomography (CT) A method of using x-rays and computer technology to show a cross-section view of the internal organs.

core biopsy A type of biopsy where the needle cuts a cylindrically shaped core from the target tissue.

cryosurgery A type of therapy that freezes the cancer cells for treatment.

cystoscopy A lighted telescope is placed into the bladder through the urethra for examination.

Digital Rectal Exam (DRE) Examination by the doctor of the rectum and prostate by inserting a gloved finger.

ejaculation The act of semen ejecting from the penis.

erectile dysfunction Inability to sustain or achieve an erection.

erection The enlargement and hardening of the penis when it becomes filled with blood.

estrogen Female hormone.

external urethral sphincter A band of muscle fibers that voluntarily contracts the passage of urine from the bladder to the outside.

Flutamide A drug taken to provide androgen blockage.

Foley catheter A thin rubber tube that is placed into the bladder so it can continously drain the urine.

foreplay Sexual activity before intercourse. Extended amount not followed by ejaculation can cause prostate congestion and irritation.

frozen section A technique in which the tissue that is removed is frozen, then cut into thin slices and stained to be examined under a microscope.

false negative An incorrect report of a test that is actually positive.

false positive An incorrect report of a test that is actually negative.

genitourinary tract the urinary system includes the kidneys, ureters, bladder, and urethra and genital system includes testicles, vas deferens, penis, and prostate gland.

gland Organ or structure that secretes a substance to be used or discharged from the body.

Gleason score A method to classify the degree of malignancy in the cells.

grade An assignment of the degree of malignancy determined by microscopic appearance of malignant cells.

groin Part of the body where the legs attach to the body at the lower part of the abdomen.

hematuria Blood in the urine.

heredity Characteristics that are handed down from parents to their children through genetic material.

hesitancy A delay in getting the urinary stream to flow.

High Density Lipoprotein (HDL) It is produced mainly in the liver and carries cholesterol away from the arteries and back to the liver. Known as good guys, as a high level seems to protect against a heart condition.

hormonal therapy Treatment for prostate cancer to block hormone production through surgery or chemical means.

hormone Those which are responsible for the development of the secondary sex characteristics.

hypertrophy The excessive growth development of an organ or part of it.

hyperthermia Heating of the prostate to destroy the prostate tissue that is causing problems.

immune system System of organs, blood cells, tissue, and substances that are able to fight off infections, cancer, and other foreign proteins that can make the person ill.

impotence The lack or inability of a man to develop or maintain an erection that is adequate for vaginal penetration.

incontinent Inability to control the flow of urine.

infection Injury to tissue caused by pathogenic microorganisms that invade the body and grow and produce toxins.

IVP (Intravenous pyelogram) X-ray pictures taken after injection of dyes intravenously into the bloodstream that allow the doctor to diagnose problems of the urinary tract.

Kegel exercises Exercises of the pelvis that help to strengthen the muscles used with urination. Helpful to overcome incontinence and sexual problems.

local anesthesia Numbs a specific area of the body prior to surgery or other form of treatment so patient will not experience pain.

local therapy Treatment that affects a tumor.

Low Density Lipoprotein (LDL) Is the major cholesterol carrier in the blood. When it has too much it can form plaque to clog the arteries and contribute to heart attack or stroke. LDL is known as the bad guys.

luteinizing hormone—releasing hormone (LHRH) A hormone that acts on the testes to stimulate testosterone production.

lymph Is an almost colorless fluid that travels through the lymphatic system and carries the cells that fight infection.

lymphatic system The tissues and organs that produce, store, and carry cells that fight infection and disease. The bone marrow, spleen, thymus, lymph nodes, and channels that carry lymph are part of this system.

lymph nodes Small bean-shaped organs throughout the body that store special cells that are able to trap bacteria or cancer cells traveling through the body in lymph. They are also referred to as lymph glands.

malignancy Cancerous, as in malignant tumor—the potential of spreading to other parts of the body.

masturbation The stimulation of the genital organs other than during intercourse.

metastasis The spread of cancer from one part of the body to another.

MRI (Magnetic Resonance Imaging) This method produces a cross-sectional image much like the cat scan. It does not use x-rays.

nocturia Awakening during the night with a desire to urinate.

nocturnal emission Commonly referred to as a wet dream, where the semen is discharged during sleep.

nuclear scan A test using radioactive trace compounds to help the doctor diagnose the problem.

oncologist Doctor who has had specialized training in the treatment of cancer.

orchiectomy Surgical operation to remove the testicles.

outpatient Surgery or treatment that does not require checking into a hospital and having to stay overnight.

pathologist A doctor who has had special training to identify diseases by studying cells and tissues under a microscope.

pelvic The area of the body located below the waist and surrounded by the hip and pubic bone.

penile Relating to the penis.

penile prosthesis A device that is surgically implanted to provide erections for men who are impotent.

perineum Area located just behind the scrotum in front of the anus.

placebo An inactive substance used as a control in an experiment. Contains no medication.

polyunsaturated and monounsaturated fatty acids Polyunsaturated and monounsaturated fatty acids make up the total of unsaturated fatty acids. They're often found in liquid oils of vegetable origin. Common sources of polyunsaturated fatty acids are safflower, sesame, and sunflower seeds, corn and soybeans, many nuts and seeds, and their oils. Canola, olive, and peanut oils and avocados are sources of monounsaturated fatty acids.

prognosis The probable outcome or course of a disease. The chance of recovery.

prostatectomy An operation to remove all parts of the prostate gland.

prostate gland A male sex gland located at the base of the bladder that produces semen.

prostate specific antigen (PSA) A protein that increases in the blood of some men who have benign prostate hyperplasia or prostate cancer. It is helpful to detect problems.

prostate surgery There are various approaches:

1) Perineal—An approach to the prostate through the perineum. Used also for treatment of BPH.

2) Retropubic—This approach is through the lower abdomen and behind the pubic bone; also used for BPH.

3) Suprapubic—An approach through the lower abdomen and through the bladder; also used for BPH.

4) Transurethral—A surgical approach through the lower abdomen and bladder used to surgically treat BPH.

prostatic acid phosphatase (PAP) An enzyme that is produced by the prostate. Its level in the blood goes up in some men who have prostate cancer. Use most popular before discovery of PSA.

prostatic massage A digital rectal procedure whereby the doctor with his index finger forcefully massages the two lateral lobes of the prostate to obtain secretions.

prostatitis An inflammation of the prostate gland that can be acute. Chronic or of a temporary nature. It can be caused by bacteria.

prostatostasis A prostate that is congested with prostate secretions that are usually due to irregular or infrequent ejaculation.

radiation therapy Treatment by a specially trained doctor who will use high energy rays from x-rays or other sources to damage cancer cells.

radical prostatectomy Operation whereby the entire prostate is removed, including the surrounding tissue and structures to eliminate cancer.

radioactive seeds Small pellets of substances that are radioactive and inserted into the prostate to kill cancer cells.

radiologist A specially trained doctor who performs and interprets various types of x-rays.

rectum The last 5 to 6 inches of the intestine leading to the anus.

remission The signs and symptoms of cancer disappear. When this occurs the disease is said to be in remission. It can be temporary or permanent.

renal scans Two-dimensional pictures used to determine the blood flow to the kidney, kidney function, and obstruction to drainage of the kidney.

resectoscope An instrument used so the doctor can see the prostate tissue while he cuts through the urethra.

retropubic prostatectomy The doctor removes by surgery the prostate through an incision in the abdomen.

scrotum The sac that contains the testicles.

semen The fluid that comes out of the penis during orgasm. It is made up of sperm from the testicles and also fluid from the prostate and other sex glands.

stage A medical term used to describe the size or quantity of the cancer, especially whether it has spread from its original site to other parts of the body.

suprapubic prostatectomy Removal by an operation of all or part of the prostate gland through an incision below the navel and above the pubic bone in the lower abdomen.

testicles The two glands that produce sperm and male hormones.

transurethral resection of the prostate An instrument is inserted through the penis to remove tissue from the prostate.

triglyceride Molecules of ordinary fat circulating in the blood. It is implicated in the destructive process of atherosclerosis.

tumor An abnormal mass of tissue.

tumor nodes metastases (TNM) A system that is used by doctors in the staging of cancer. The T stands for tumor. The N for lymph node involvement and the M for metastases. The number that follows the letter indicates the size of the tumor, the extent of lymph node involvement, and the extent of metastatic disease.

ultrasound Sound waves used to produce pictures of areas inside the body. They are created by a computer that interprets the echoes produced by the waves as they bounce off tissue.

urethra The tube that carries urine or semen outside the body.

urologist A physician who specializes in diseases of the urinary organs in female and the urinary and sex organs in males.

vasectomy An operation to cut off or tie the tiny tubes that brings the sperm from the testicles to the prostate gland, thus causing sterility.

Selected Bibliography

The following list of references represents approximately half of the sources used in the development of this book; these have been selected for notation based on their specific relevance to prostate-related health issues.

BOOKS

Baggish, Jeff. *Making the Prostate Therapy Decision.* Chicago: Contemporary Books, 1995.

De Vita, Vincent T., Hellman, Samuel, and Rosenberg, Steven A., eds. *Cancer: Principles and Practice of Oncology*, 2 ed. Philadelphia: J. B. Uppincott Company, 1985.

Donaldson, N. *How Did They Die?* New York: St. Martin's Press, 1980.

Fer, Mehmet F., et al. *Poorly Differentiated Neoplasms and Tumor of Unknown Origin.* Orlando, Fla: Grune & Stratton, 1986.

Haskell, Charles M., ed. *Cancer Treatment.* Philadelphia: W.B. Saunders Company, 1985.

Rous, Stephen N. *The Prostate Book: Sound Advice on Symptoms and Treatment.* New York: W.W. Norton Co., 1995.

ARTICLES AND STUDIES

Albertsen, Peter C., et al. "Long Term Survival Among Men with Conservatively Treated Localized Prostate Cancer." *Journal of the American Medical Association* (August 25/30, 1995): 626.

Armstrong, B., and Doll, R. "Environmental Factors and Cancer Incidence and Mortality in Different Countries with Special References to Dietary Practices." *International Journal of Cancer* (1975: no. 15): 617–31.

Barry, Michael J. "Watchful Waiting: Preoperative Guidance for Men Facing Prostatectomy." *Medical Aspects of Human Sexuality* (December 1989): 30.

Blasko, J.C., et al. "Organ Preservation in the Management of Carcinoma of the Prostate." *Seminars in Radiation Oncology* (October 1993): 240–49.

Blasko, John. "Radioisotope Implants Are Effective in Controlling Advanced, Localized Prostate Cancer." *COPE*, (September/October 1995).

Blute, Michael L., et al. "Transurethral Microwave Thermotherapy for Management of Benign Prostatic Hyperplasia: Results of the United States Prostatron Cooperative Study." *Journal of Urology* (November 1993): 1591–96.

Catalona, William J. "Measurement of Prostate Specific Antigen as a Screening Test for Prostate Cancer." *New England Journal of Medicine* (April 25, 1991): 324.

Chodak, Gerald W., et al. "Results of Conservative Management of Clinically Localized Prostate Cancer." *New England Journal of Medicine* (January 27, 1994): 242–48.

Chodak, G.W. "The Role of Watchful Waiting in the Management of Localized Prostate Cancer." *Cancer* (October 1, 1994): 2178–81.

Crawford, E. David, et al. "The Effect of Digital Rectal Examination on Prostate Specific Antigen Levels." *Journal of the American Medical Association* (April 22, 1992): 2227.

Cunha, Burke A., et al. "Prostatitis Hurts: Managing Prostatitis in the Elderly." *Geriatrics* (January 1991): 60.

Daniell, Harry W. "More Stage A Prostatic Cancers, Less Surgery for Benign Hypertophy in Smokers." *Journal of Urology* (January 1993): 68–72.

Dugan, James A., et al. "The Definition and Preoperative Prediction of Clinically Insignificant Prostate Cancer." *Journal of the American Medical Association* (January 24, 1996): 288.

Faiulson, Saralle. "Two Studies Link Vasectomies and Prostate Cancer but Experts Disagree." *Medical Tribune* (March 11, 1993).

Fawzy, Ahmed, et al. "Doxazosin in the Treatment of Benign Prostatic Hyperplasia in Normotensive patients, a Multi-Center Study." *Journal of Urology* (July 1995): 105–09.

Fleming, Craig, et al. "A Decision Analysis of Alternative Treatment Strategies for Clinically Localized Prostate Cancer," *Journal of the American Medical Association* (May 26, 1993): 2650–58.

Gambert, Steven R. "The Crucial Prostate Exam." *Emergency Medicine* (June 30, 1992): 25.

Gann, Peter H., et al. "A New Study Confirms Value of PSA: A Prospective Evaluation of Plasma Prostate Specific Antigen for Detection of Prostatic Cancer." *Journal of the American Medical Association* (January 1995): 289–294.

Giovannucci, E., et al. "A Prospective Cohort Study of Vasectomy and Prostate Cancer in U.S. Men," *Journal of the American Medical Association* (February 1993): 873–82.

Giovannucci, E., et al. "A Prospective Study of Dietary Fat and Risk of Prostate Cancer in U.S. Men." *Journal of the National Cancer Institute* (October 6, 1993): 1571.

Giovannucci, E., et al. "Intake of Carotenoids and Retinol in Relation to Risk of Prostate Cancer." *Journal of the National Cancer Institute* (December 6, 1995): 1571–79.

Gittes, R.F., "Carcinoma of the Prostate (10-Year Summary)," *New England Journal of Medicine* (January 24, 1991): 236–45.

Goldbalm, A. Alexandra, et al. "Consumption of Black Tea and Cancer Risk: A Prospective Cohort Study." *Journal of the National Cancer Institute* (January 17, 1996): 93–100.

Henderan, B.B. "Countries That Have High Fat Diets: Summary Report of the Sixth Symposium on Cancer Registries and Epidemiology in the Pacific Basin." *Journal of the National Cancer Institute* (July 18, 1990): 1186–90.

Hennekens, Charles, and Buring, Julie E. "Anti-Oxidants." *New England Journal of Medicine* (Vol. 330, No. 15): 180.

Jacobson, Steven E., et al. "Incidence of Prostate Cancer Diagnosis in the Eras Before and After Serum Prostate Specific Antigen Testing." *Journal of the American Medical Association* (November 1995): 1445.

Jenkins, E.P. et al. "Genetic and Pharmacological Evidence for More Than One Human Steroid 5 Alpha Reductase." *Journal of Clinical Investigation* (January 1992): 293–300.

Johansson, Jan-Erick, et al. "High Ten Year Survival Rate in Patients with Early Untreated Prostatic Cancer." *Journal of the American Medical Association* (April 22/29, 1992): 2191–96.

John, Esther M., et al. "Vasectomy and Prostate Cancer: Results from a Multiethnic Case Control Study." *Journal of the National Cancer Institute* (May 3, 1995): 662.

Klamet, Anita, et al. "Community Prostate Cancer Screening." *Cancer Practice* (November/December 1995): 366.

Lee, I.M. "Physical Activity and Risk of Prostate Cancer Among College Alumni." *American Journal of Epidemiology* (Vol. 135, no. 2): 169–79.

Lu-Yao, Grace L., et al. "An Assessment of Radical Prostatectomy: Time Trends, Geographic Variation, and Outcomes." *Journal of the American Medical Association* (May 1993): 2633–36.

Lu-Yao, G.L., et al. "Transurethral Resection of the Prostate Among Medicare Beneficiaries in the United States: Time Trends and Outcomes." *Urology* (November 1994): 692–99.

Mann, Charles C. "The Prostate Dilemma." *Atlantic Monthly* (November 1993): 118.

McCann, Jean. "Microwaving Prostate Problems Away: Geriatric Consultation." *The Partnership of Academia and Industry in Pharmacologic Research* (May/June 1992): 21.

McWharter, William P., et al. "A Screening Study of Prostate Cancer in High Risk Families." *Journal of Urology* (September 1992): 826–28.

Morrow, Alan S. "Difference in Race Risk Factors for Prostate Hypertrophy." *American Journal of Epidemiology* (November 1992).

Novelli, Lynn. "PSA Screens: A Hole in the Theory." *Modern Medicine* (July 1993).

Oesterling, Joseph E., et al. "The Use of Prostate Specific Antigen in Staging Patients with Newly Diagnosed Prostate Cancer." *Journal of the American Medical Association* (January 6, 1993): 57–60.

Peters, Craig A., and Walsh, Patrick C. "The Effect of Nafarelin Acetate, a Luteinizing Hormone Agonist, on Benign Prostatic Hyperplasia." *New England Journal of Medicine* (September 1987): 599.

Phaleon, Richard. "Eleven Options." *Forbes* (August 17, 1992): 118.

Pisters, Louis L., and Babaian, Richard. "Evaluating Screening Tools for Prostatic Cancer." *Hospital Medicine* (November 1993): 62.

Ross, R.K., and Henderson, B.E. "Segments of Population at Risk: Do Diet and Androgen Alter Prostate Cancer Risk Via a Common Etiologic Pathway?" *Journal of the National Cancer Institute* (February 1994): 252.

Scardino, Peter T. "Early Diagnosis of Prostate Cancer Vital to Cure the Disease." *Urology's Clinical Research and Socioeconomic Newspaper* (September 1991).

Stamey, Thomas A. "Early Detection of Prostate Cancer: A Guide to Screening." *American Urological Association Today* (September 1991): 4–11.

Stamey, Thomas A., et al. "Prostate Specific Antigen as a Serum Marker for Adenocarcinoma of the Prostate." *New England Journal of Medicine* (October 8, 1987): 909–16.

Takayama, M.D., and Lange, Paul H. "Radiation Therapy for Local Recurrence of Prostate Cancer and Radical Prostatectomy." *Urologic Clinics of North America* (November 1994): 687.

Tchetgen, Marie-Blanche, et al. "Influence of Patient Age on the Serum Prostate-Specific Antigen." *Urologic Clinics of North America* (1993, No. 4): 671–79.

Thingpea, A.E., et al. "Briff Report: The Molecular Basis of Steroid 5 Alpha Reductase Deficiency in a Large Dominican Kindred." *New England Journal of Medicine* (1992, No. 327): 1216–19.

Walsh, P.C., and Donker, P.J. "Impotence Following a Radical Prostatectomy: Insight into Etiology and Prevention." *Journal of Urology* (September 1982): 492–97.

Walsh, P.C. "Prostate Cancer Increasing: Prostate Cancer Kills Strategy to Reduce Deaths." Paper presented at the American Urological Association Meeting (May 1994).

White, Ralph deVere, et al. "Urinary Prostate Specific Antigen Levels: Role in Monitoring the Response of Prostate Cancer to Therapy." *Journal of Urology* (March 1992): 947–951.

Whitmore, W.F., et al. "Conservative Management of Localized Prostatic Cancer." *American Journal of Clinical Oncology* (Vol. 15, No. 5): 446–52.

Whitmore, W.F., et al. "Expectant Management of Localized Prostate Cancer." *Cancer* (Febuary 15, 1991): 1091–96.

Whittmore, Alice S., et al. "Prostate Cancer in Relation to Diet, Physical Activity and Body Size in Blacks, Whites and Asians in the U.S. and Canada." *Journal of the National Cancer Institute* (May 3, 1995): 652.

Index

A

D

Q

R

S